# TAKING CONTROL

## My Journey of Alternative Healing

Alyssia Sade

authorHOUSE®

*AuthorHouse™ UK Ltd.*
*1663 Liberty Drive*
*Bloomington, IN 47403 USA*
*www.authorhouse.co.uk*
*Phone: 0800.197.4150*

*Published by AuthorHouse 03/07/2014*

*ISBN: 978-1-4918-9748-5 (sc)*
*ISBN: 978-1-4918-9747-8 (hc)*
*ISBN: 978-1-4918-9749-2 (e)*

To Perry, the man I love. You are my soul mate; we have been through so much together. Without you, I would not know how to carry on.

To all the countless men and women who I have met whilst on this journey who have healed themselves or a loved one with alternative cures and had the tenacity to commit to it 100 per cent and then document everything and put out their testimonies for others to read and be inspired. Without you, all we have achieved would have been impossible.

To my sons and their wives for their unconditional love and support in our decision not to undergo radical surgery, chemo, and radiation and, instead, opt for a gentler way to heal.

# CONTENTS

Chapter 1   Diagnosis that Would Change
            Our Lives Forever. . . . . . . . . . . . . . . . . . . . . . . . 1
Chapter 2   A Terrible Silence. . . . . . . . . . . . . . . . . . . . . . . 6
Chapter 3   Choosing Alternative Therapy over
            Conventional Poison. . . . . . . . . . . . . . . . . . . . . .11
Chapter 4   Coping with Disappointment . . . . . . . . . . . . . . . . 33
Chapter 5   Difficult Decisions . . . . . . . . . . . . . . . . . . . . . . 43
Chapter 6   Laser Surgery . . . . . . . . . . . . . . . . . . . . . . . . . 75
Chapter 7   An Illegal Treatment. . . . . . . . . . . . . . . . . . . . . 77
Chapter 8   Dark Months . . . . . . . . . . . . . . . . . . . . . . . . . 97
Chapter 9   Dissapointment. . . . . . . . . . . . . . . . . . . . . . . .115
Chapter 10  Renewed Hope . . . . . . . . . . . . . . . . . . . . . . . .117
Chapter 11  Looking Back. . . . . . . . . . . . . . . . . . . . . . . . .136

# PREFACE

*I am married to the most amazing man, who I'll be calling Perry throughout* Taking Control. *"Perry" and I have three sons, and we've recently been blessed with two beautiful granddaughters. Because we live and work in the Middle East, I've changed all the names in our story and am writing under the pseudonym Alyssia Sade'. However, the dates and all other information in* Taking Control *are a true account of the nineteen months from July 2012, when Perry was first diagnosed with cancer, through January 2014, when we confirmed for the second time that he was cancer free, and the journey we undertook in order to heal him naturally.*

I would never be so bold as to tell someone to change the way he or she thinks or to do anything he or she doesn't wholeheartedly believe in. But I will ask you to open your minds to new beliefs. If you have any doubt about what chemotherapy and radiation will do to your body, then perhaps it is time to research what can aid your own body's natural healing power. The human body is an amazing machine, and all we need to do to keep it running that way is to feed it the right nutrition.

Fear is a terrible thing, and fear is ripe when we hear the word *cancer*. The phrase *frightened to death* is really what happens to the body once you believe there is only one way to treat this terrible disease.

I hope that sharing my journal might give the reader at least some hope that there is another way. Our belief system does not have to be locked. We can open up our minds to think for ourselves, inform ourselves, and learn not to just accept our "fate".

# FOREWORD

## by Robin Swan

Between 2005 and 2007, nine of my family members died from various forms of cancer. Throughout my career, I had worked with and buried too many women who had suffered and lost the battle to breast cancer.

As a holistic health practitioner who has spent a lifetime learning about alternative forms of healing, I was at a loss as to what to do. I had been raised in the cannabis industry, and I was well aware of all of the medicinal components of the plant for things like glaucoma and depression and nausea. My grandmothers and aunties had been making tincture and balms with the plant materials for my entire life. I had continued these traditions and always offered the tinctures and balms to my clients, but they weren't enough. It helped ease the pain but could not stop the suffering and death. At my mother's funeral, one of my cousins asked me if I had heard of a man named Rick Simpson in Canada. He was extracting the plant in a way that had not been done since 4000 BC. I had not, and I immediately set about finding out everything I could about this man and his extraction process. This led to many conversations via email with Rick and reading his books and watching parts of the film *Run from the Cure* hundreds of times. I was hungry for something to bring back to my world that would actually change the direction and course of this heinous disease. Rick's methodology offered me a new direction—a way of processing the plant that kept the molecular structure intact. I learned we all had something called the endocannabinoid system in our bodies that was interlocking with our brains and that ingesting the plant this way activated that system and not only repaired the myelin sheath of the nerve; the THC actually ate the tumours! This seemed miraculous! What if it was true? What if it worked?

A truth about human beings is that we'll do whatever is necessary to help and prolong the life of someone we love. We will travel to the ends of the earth and spend our last dollar on magic beans if we believe it will heal our beloved. There is no risk too great to take if it means we will get just one more day with whomever we love. Being filled with compassion for this process my partner and I decided it was time to do our part.

We took our love of the plant and all our years as herbalists and growers, and we began creating the most powerful example of what Rick Simpson was sharing and what has been recorded truth all the way back to the ancient Sarmatians, repeating itself over and over again throughout history on every continent and in most cultures. We made cannabis concentrate and started to share it.

The first batch went to a client who had been living with breast cancer for twelve years. She had kept it at bay with many different forms of chemo, radiation, diet, and whatever else medicinal and herbal science had to offer. She was hopeful but not convinced. But medical science had given up on her, and she was sent home to live out whatever time she had left.

After using the oil for just a few months, the cancer had completely disappeared the tumours were gone. Her doctors were amazed, and she was, for the first time in over a decade, healed and pronounced cancer free!

We knew we were onto the truth and continued feeding the oil to my clients. No one knew of this remedy at the time, and the learning curve was great! Hours were spent educating that, yes, this was "pot"; however, it wasn't a drug for deadbeat losers who live in their parent's basements—it was a remedy that was over 4,000 years old.

Because of the legality of it, people were somewhat unresponsive to it. This was more than frustrating for me. Here I was offering this amazing form of medicine, using the oldest most versatile plant on the planet, and because of the law, people were afraid to use it. Those who took the risk did amazing!

After much soul searching, I decided it was time to share our experiences with the populous of the world. It wasn't important to me that doing so might land me in jail. Rick had paved the way, and many warriors had gone down in this battle to save lives. The good of many outweighed the good of the one. I decided that the best avenue for this was Facebook. I would take the risk and share my stories with the world, using the fastest vehicle I knew available—social media.

Within hours of me posting pictures of my clients and their success stories, I was getting thousands of hits! Inboxes messages were pouring in! I was amazed—and encouraged by my attorney to stop doing it!

Stopping wasn't an option. So many people were at their wits' end. My partner and I decided to donate a few pounds of plant material, and we set about sending out free samples to anyone who inquired. The response was astronomical! There is no shortage of people who will go to the end of the earth to find a thread of hope for someone they love. The open-hearted response from the world was humbling and overwhelming. The responsibility became immense. The need for the healing power of this plant

We the people wanted to return to what was growing naturally on our planet and to what, for all of recorded human history, has been used for food, shelter, clothing, and medicine. The most sacred plant on the planet was reawakening.

Through this blossoming of knowledge, I met Alyssia and Perry. They were already on the right track. She had done all of her research, and Perry was on board with one of the most important pieces of treating any body imbalance—correct nutrition. During one of our Skype conversations, Alyssia shared with me that she had been keeping a journal. She invited me to read it. She was my first client who had been keeping track of the progress and how-to of treatment. I was very excited and not at all let down when I read it and saw her artwork.

I encouraged her to publish this journal because it was a very timely story filled with everything all people go through when they are looking for a cure, an alternative approach. The journal breaks down many aspects of healing this disease. The truth of our human struggle is balanced with how we need to feed our machine.

There is no one answer for what cures cancer. There is only what works consistently for most people. A body of work like this defines hope by giving it structure. It shows us a way to implement a healing path. Alyssia answers so many questions in this journal. If you or a loved one is living with cancer, this is a must-read. If you're considering an alternative medicine, such as cannabis oil, this is a must-read. It is our faith in each other that creates hope and offers up our charitable wholehearted selves in an act of love. May this book assist you on your personal path to the richest disease-free life available to you.

Love all, serve all,
Robin Swan

# CHAPTER 1

## DIAGNOSIS THAT WOULD CHANGE OUR LIVES FOREVER

### July 2012

Whilst on a trip back to England, my husband, Perry, was suffering a terrible backache, which had been niggling him for some ten weeks by this time. He was in so much pain that we returned home early to visit the doctor back in the Middle East, where we lived and worked.

The doctors had first thought the pain was just sciatica all those weeks ago. He had seen quite a few doctors, but he'd found no relief. He was prescribed very strong painkillers, which helped to ease the discomfort slightly. On this visit, though, the doctor gave him a pain injection, as the pain had gotten worse. But within hours, Perry noticed that his urine had turned a deep brown colour. We thought this had to be a reaction to the pain injection, so we left it to see if it cleared. When it continued the next morning, I was very concerned; I thought that he might have blood in his urine. So we scheduled an appointment yet again.

Perry had a CT scan on his bladder, which showed something small in the bladder. The doctor told us he thought this might be a kidney stone and that it might just pass by itself. But when the blood came back, the doctor realized that the initial complaint of backache had to take a back seat, as something more urgent than his back problems needed to be investigated.

He was referred to a local specialist urologist; after having some additional urine testing, he met with the urologist.

During our first appointment, the specialist looked at the scans and informed us very matter-of-factly "it could be a tumour."

He softened the blow by adding that it could be benign like a cyst. But to be sure he needed to do a cystoscopy. He noted that 99 per cent of the time, a person Perry's age with this issue would be just fine and that we probably just needed to make sure.

We were moving through various stages of feelings. And I was reading as much as I could. I was really quite concerned by this time but tried not to let my worry show.

## August 2012

My husband was diagnosed with bladder cancer.

The surgeon urologist had told me that my husband would be in surgery for just thirty minutes. He had assured me that, with his twenty-five years of experience in this field, he would be able to see whether what was *plaguing Perry's body* was cancer and that he would be able to tell us straight away if it wasn't; he assured me it would be a standard quick procedure. My youngest son was with a friend and also me; we were so laid-back about the outcome, my son and friend left me and said they would come back later with some food, as Perry would be hungry when he woke.

Thirty minutes passed very slowly and still no sign of the doctor. Then, over an hour later, he came to the waiting room doorway to inform me that he could not do the biopsy properly, as he could not see clearly enough. He told me he only had a window of around thirty seconds before there was too much blood for him to do the cystectomy properly. But he took slices for biopsy, and we'd just have to wait to see what the pathology lab came back with. I reminded him that he had promised me that, relying on his twenty-five years of experience, he would let me know what he thought right away, and so he told me.

From what he could see, it was definitely cancer; not only that, it was a very aggressive and invasive form of cancer. He added that he had seen more than one tumour but could not be sure how many were there as there was too much blood. Perry's bladder, the doctor explained, was like a mass of jellied blood.

At that moment, I felt my world turn upside down. All kinds of thoughts flashed in my head at the same time. I was trying to keep myself upright; I felt faint, sick, and about to pass out. I was not prepared to hear this terrible news at all.

I could hear him still talking, something about how I shouldn't tell my husband, as he had to recover from the surgery, and how he would have a plan of action to present to him once he got the exact stage of the cancer.

Thoughts rushed through my mind all at once, and all I could envisage was that I was going to lose him—the love of my life and the man I had been married to for thirty-three years. *Shock* was not a strong enough word; it was as if my very soul was being sucked out of my body. I was shaking. I wanted to get the food I had just eaten out of my body; it began to weigh heavy in my stomach, and I knew I would not keep it down for much longer.

I could not take it in. I didn't know what to do. My husband's colleague from work had visited and decided to stay with me until Perry came out of recovery. I could see him watching the look on my face as I was speaking with the surgeon. I needed to be alone so I could let go of all this pent-up emotion. I went to the bathroom in the waiting room and let out a guttural scream. It was as if that cry had come from somewhere else. There was no air. I could hardly breathe. Terror such as I had never before felt consumed me. After throwing up, I somehow ended up sitting on the bathroom floor rocking myself back and forth for some time. A nurse was in the bathroom cleaning her teeth, and she just carried on as if I wasn't even there. And so I carried on, letting out all of my hurt right in front of her.

I then realized that, if I did not stop crying and sort myself out, Perry would know something was very wrong. I had to get control of myself so I could help him recover from this surgery.

All I wanted was to call our older sons in England, and I couldn't get hold of them. The lady anaesthetist who had been with us both earlier had enjoyed seeing us both laugh and joke before he went down to surgery. She'd asked how many cigarettes he smoked, and I had answered thirty as Perry had said ten. She'd smiled while writing thirty on his paperwork. We'd joked with her about how long we had been married.

Now she came to me, put her hand on my arm, and said not to worry; he would be out soon. She clearly could see how upset I was and asked if I had family here. I told her my older sons were in England, and she informed me that she thought it would be a good idea for me to ask them to come to me! *I panicked, my hysteria still clearly not under control. "He's going to die now?" I blurted out.*

She assured me that she meant she thought I needed someone here to support me too. She asked me to dry my eyes and just try to be brave for Perry so that he could get well from his surgery—that it was best not to tell him the full extent of his condition yet

I made a decision there and then that I hope I have fulfilled—to do this with as much grace and dignity, as I could muster. I kept a brave face. But when the attendants wheeled him out of the operating room, I kissed him passionately leaving my face on his for as long as I could.

I told him I had just been so worried about him and that he had been in the operating room for much longer than we'd thought he would be. He kept asking me what was wrong.

I stayed in the hospital for three days and nights, not sleeping or eating, wondering how long I would have my precious husband. I let our sons know what I knew, but keeping it all from the one person I should have no secrets from was extremely difficult. I watched him eating and laughing at the television without a care in the world, and it broke my heart.

Perry's boss came to the hospital with the same colleague who'd been with me earlier. Even they knew about the diagnosis before he did. His boss sat and laughed and joked with us, but secretly he'd come to offer me any support I might need.

We returned home, but many secret phone calls to family and friends in the UK were made. My husband's brother called Perry in the hospital and expressed how upset he was. Though my brother-in-law had been told that his brother did not know anything about the cancer yet, he told Perry that his sister had gone to him and they had both cried together. I was so angry with my brother-in-law; at this time as I was trying to hold it together for my husband's sake; the least he could do was do the same. I had to lie to my husband then, saying I had no idea why his brother would be so upset; perhaps he just could not bear the thought of him being so far away and in hospital.

# CHAPTER 2
## A TERRIBLE SILENCE

Five days after the surgery, we had the appointment with the urologist. We learned that Perry's cancer was invasive, stage T2, and the plan the doctor advised included removing his bladder, prostate, and some lymph nodes. He told us a neo bladder could be fashioned from Perry's intestines, but it would be better to go home to our own country for the operation, as a team of doctors would be needed.

I had told my husband the night before we had the appointment that the tumour had been cancerous, as I could not let a stranger deliver this news.

I didn't know then that we had options, but what I did know is that I owed it to myself, and my husband to do my damnedest to find out.

Once I had a purpose, it gave my thoughts direction. By the time we left hospital, I had already started all my research. I first looked at the best hospitals for this type of surgery. We had no knowledge of cancer or chemo other than what I had seen on the television. I'd never had any family members have this dreadful disease. I thought the only option would be to find the best surgeons and, first, to get a second opinion. So we immediately flew to England.

We both hoped there had been some terrible mistake, and we needed to go to our own country to talk to experts without a language barrier. My husband, still in a state of shock, was terribly quiet; he did not speak to me the whole of the long flight home.

Family members wanted to meet us at the airport, but we did not want to face them yet. We had to keep it together, and them crying would not help. So we decided to go straight to a hotel and then the hospital.

Within another few days, Perry had his second biopsy. The specialist urologist had performed Lady Archer's bladder removal, a fact that he was very proud of and that had been mentioned in all the national press outlets. I felt a little comforted at this point; we had at least found a great surgeon. We returned to the home of our family members we were staying with, until the biopsy results were ready. With everyone running around trying to be of some help but ending up crying and feeling sorry for us. This waiting period was really hard.

Perry was withdrawing into a terrible silence. One day, he wouldn't even get out of bed. He refused to talk to anyone and just wanted to be left alone. Those few days, as we waited to hear his fate, were the worst days of our entire journey along the path that would eventually tell us his fate.

We returned to Cambridge, about an hour away from our hometown, and decided to stay in a hotel again the night before we were to meet with the surgeon again. During the entire drive to the hotel, Perry was silent and on throughout the night. It was agonizing.

The surgeon (who was emotionless and looked like an undertaker) informed us that the cancer was indeed invasive, as the first biopsy had proved, and not only did the surgical team need to remove his bladder, prostate and possibly lymph nodes, they also recommend that he do six rounds of chemotherapy beforehand; they had now staged the cancer as T2A—invading the muscle wall. This, he explained, was far more serious than first suspected.

Bacillus Chalmette-Guerin (BCG), a treatment that entailed the medicine of the tuberculosis vaccine, which was known to kill cancer cells, whilst leaving the good cells to thrive, couldn't treat it. BCG was designed for superficial bladder cancer, a carcinoma in situ. The cancer can't spread elsewhere, as the cancer cells haven't broken through the membrane of the growth. The doctor also informed us, "The factory that made the vaccine had been closed due to a flood." So even if this were an option, the hospital would not be able to get it!

He suggested that we first go to see an oncologist about the chemo; *I wouldn't realize until later that the urologist and the oncologist worked together regularly, sharing patients, and that chemotherapy was an important moneymaker for their private practice.*

The Oncologist suggested we do the chemo before the operation. But I had been researching ever since we'd first found out that chemotherapy might be a recommendation, and I'd learned about many people having gone through chemotherapy and dying because of it. He offered radiation too, but I'd also found out that many people have to be treated for the burns they receive during radiation therapy.

We had a few days before we were to visit the surgeon again. He stressed that, with the surgery, chemo, and radiation, there was a very good chance of a total cure. We asked how long Perry would have to live if we did nothing. We were told one to two years at the most.

We returned to our hometown to have some time to think about things. My brother offered us his house, where we could be alone. We were going back and forth in our minds about what we should do—take the surgery or live the one to two years the best way we could, together and happy. Alone in my thoughts, I imagined never being able to make love again with this man I adored; I was consumed with my own grief. Our lovemaking was wild and passionate, as if it was going to be the last time. We were, I suppose, in effect saying goodbye to this part of our lives in preparation. I knew all along that, if the time came, I would go with him. I told him so too. I vowed to take some tablets and feed them to him as well before the end came, and I meant every word.

After we'd had a few days alone together, we decided we needed some more time to let all this terrible news sink in and to look into whether we had any options. Everyone was upset and feeling sorry for us. It was all too much to take in, and we couldn't come to the right decision in just a few days.

We spoke again to the urologist and told him we needed more time to research alternative treatments and modalities. We would not take the chemo just yet. We explained that we were already looking into different therapies and that both of us were concerned with the quality of his life after surgery. We needed time to digest all of this dreadful news.

The oncologist and the surgeon both tried to impress on us that we needed to think very carefully about the surgery. The surgeon had already set a date in his schedule to proceed with the bladder removal. We felt like we were being railroaded into this far too quickly, and we needed to slow this train down a little so we could have time to digest everything. Something was screaming at me to take some time before making this radical decision.

I felt completely alone as I struggled to figure out how we could save my husband's bladder while also saving his life. The doctors weren't helping us in any way when they told us that Perry's only chance was to remove his bladder, in the hope the cancer would not spread to other organs. The surgeon even tried to frighten us with graphic details of how painful a death it would be if the cancer did spread to other organs, adding that is what would happen if we didn't remove his bladder as soon as possible. He did this once he'd realized we weren't going to sign anything that would commit Perry to the operation right then and there. He was probably thinking of his yearly quota!

I'd researched what this operation did to a man, and I couldn't let this happen to Perry. The doctor never went into the details of the pain and suffering he would endure—the incontinence and infections this operation would bring. He didn't mention that the entire operation, including building a neo bladder, could take up to a year of recovery, if he recovered at all, without infections. Neither did he say anything of the fact that Perry would be rendered impotent.

I felt sure there was something more we could do; there had to be! Perry was just fifty-two years old; we were still in love; he was at the top of his career; and we had so much we still wanted to see and do. We had a wonderful life together. I was screaming inside for some answers, all the while researching every waking moment.

The research about bladder removal scared me to death, and I couldn't discuss it with Perry at this time. It was all too fresh, and he had too much to deal with at the moment, just being diagnosed. God only knew how hard this was for him to deal with. He had no idea what his prognosis would be if he were to go ahead with the operation. He only knew that, if he did nothing, he would have eighteen months or so to live. He was doing no research at all. I was doing all of it while he tried to come to terms with what he would have to deal with and get well after his second biopsy in just two weeks. Yes he may survive cancer, but what would be his quality of life? Even the doctor told us this operation was usually performed on a seventy-year-old man.

# CHAPTER 3

## CHOOSING ALTERNATIVE THERAPY OVER CONVENTIONAL POISON

We went back to speak with our sons. We discussed with them what the doctor had said and told them we were considering not doing the operation at all. Perry informed them that he would rather take the two years than live like an old man. I told them we were looking into whether we had any other options—that we wouldn't just do nothing, but we needed to find out what we could do other than the removal of these vital organs.

England no longer felt like home to us, as we had been abroad for nearly twelve years. We needed to go back to the place we knew as home; we needed space and to be in our own surroundings while we figured things out.

Our oldest son told us of a friend of his, whose wife had taken an alternative medicine called Essiac for breast cancer and who was willing to talk to us about their decision to go with alternative therapies. Our two older sons and their wives all agreed they would support and respect our decision not to do the operation, chemo, or radiation

Essiac a natural cancer cure, was named for Rene Caisse (the last name spelled backwards) a Canadian nurse who promoted this herbal remedy from the 1920s through the 1070's I started researching it immediately. This herbal cure consisted of four main herbs that grow in the wilderness of Ontario, Canada. The original formula was believed to have its roots from the native Canadian Ojibwa Indians. The four main herbs that make up Essiac are burdock root, slippery elm inner bark, sheep sorrel, and Indian rhubarb root.

To learn more about Rene Caisse's, "Immune System Theory" in her own words, Google "Rene Caisse story". Far too many stories and testimonials of this amazing healing medicine working on many cancers exist for me to include them here, but I urge everyone to do his or her own research.

After hours and hours of research, Perry and I decided to get some Essiac in the form of a tincture. My husband started this herbal treatment right away and, as of 18 September 2012, (five weeks after his diagnosis) had been on this for three weeks.

★　★　★

We flew back home to the Middle East, knowing we had to give this medicine at least six weeks to work. Then we'd try to get the urologist here to check and see whether the cancer was regressing or if, as the surgeons had predicted, it had progressed. We were warned that we should not wait longer than six to eight weeks before starting the chemotherapy. We were worried, as we had no knowledge of our own; we simply had to trust what these genius doctors were telling us. The surgeon in the UK had told us that the last biopsy had removed 90 per cent of the tumour but it would grow back rapidly if we did nothing, and in his professional opinion, Perry should have six cycles of chemotherapy right away. He said we couldn't delay for longer than four to six weeks.

Getting back to our own home and our own surroundings was very calming. It seemed like life had gone back to normal. Perry concentrated on getting back to work, while I researched every minute I had. I was blessed not to have to go out to work. I am an artist so can work when I feel like it, I had all the time I needed.

My daughter-in-law had given me a book about a woman who cured her own cancer through a process, sort of regression and meditation. "The Journey" written by Brandon Bays, was very powerful and deeply moving to me. I read her book from cover to cover to my husband on car journeys, in waiting rooms at the doctors' offices, and while he was in hospital. I couldn't put it down. It was the beginning of both my husband's and my own spiritual journey. I've encouraged all of my friends and loved ones to read this book. It moved me to tears and gave me the courage like I saw in its author and a sense of calm.

I wanted to try to get in touch with Brandon, as like she had, I also had a deep sixth sense that there was a reason my husband had the cancer growing inside him and if we could find the reason then we would find the cure. I knew already that deeply routed issues were the cause of most illnesses, and I had my own suspicions to what was causing my husband's cancer. But I'll not share the details here, as they're deeply personal: What I do want share, is all the alternative routes we would take and our experiences of them.

My daughter-in-law located a practitioner of the Journeywork Brandon taught in her book, who practiced in the country we live. I called her right away and explained the situation. She asked if my husband was interested, and he said he was open to trying anything.

He had one session with her, and he was convinced she had cured him of cancer. He was calm and obviously still looking at other alternative treatments, but he felt that something was going on, on the inside. He had opened up to her in her session about things that were very deeply rooted. He'd thought they were insignificant, but they'd come up in the session, and he'd gotten rid of them with her help.

Just by chance, a friend of mine told us about the Fuda Cancer Hospital in China. We had not realized how many alternatives were available to us, and we were opening up so much information. It was enlightening and also frightening that there are so many alternative cures for cancer. We both researched this clinic night and day and then decided to send the hospital the medical records. They were immediate in their response and assured us that they could treat the cancer with immunotherapy, without removing the bladder. Immunotherapy builds the immune system and does not destroy it, like conventional Western cancer treatments do.

We were soon in the process of acquiring visas and the okay from our insurance company. But we ran into a snag when our insurer declared that not enough data supported immunotherapy as a viable treatment for them to pay for. At this point, we had the invitation letter from the hospital. All we needed to do was go to the Chinese Embassy to apply for the visas. Once we had the go-ahead from the insurance company, we could book the tickets and room at the hospital. It was all happening so quickly.

My faith assured me that, whatever the outcome of our journey, I had nothing to fear. It was ultimately in God's hands, and all I could really ask for was the strength to get through this together.

I must say though that I was stunned at the wide variety of choices of non-toxic, gentle cancer treatments, each of which had been documented and proven to have healed cancers for thousands of people and all of them at a much higher success rates than conventional chemotherapy or radiation.

Every day, I marvelled at the politics and greed that drives our medical system and its massive cost in human lives. I would never have known this if it weren't for my husband's diagnosis. I was fast becoming aware that each of us is blessed with the opportunity to save ourselves, or our loved ones, from cancer or its treatment (usually the latter). I'd researched survivors and their testimonies and had read hundreds of them from all over the world! They all shared a common passion for finding an alternative—and we were certainly going to follow their example. They were all very positive about their future and their ability to cope with the cancer much better than they would if they were following the standard treatment. They had all taken charge of their own health care. (In other words, they didn't just "trust their doctors".) They had the mental and physical discipline to follow a regimen for an extended period of time (actually to change their lifestyles).

Most had used a variety of substances and treatments to get their cancer under control. Rarely did they rely on one substance or treatment and succeed in long-term survival.

They had found a medical professional to monitor their recovery that they trust to co-doctor with them.

They had an "advocate" (spouse, friend, or relative) who shared their recovery effort.

I now strongly believed that the free exploring mind of every individual was our most valuable asset, and the more I researched, the more I was shocked to learn that natural cures for cancer were available. And if we were to just listen to our doctors without informing ourselves, we could quickly be led down a very grave path. Where else would we go to find these cures but the Internet? I would cure my husband's bladder cancer myself, with the help of the Internet and an enquiring mind that is passionate and relentless about finding the answer.

In the book *World without Cancer*, I discovered what causes cancer and the simple ways to stop and or prevent it. For three weeks, I researched page after page from cancer journals, lectures, and individual testimonies. I wondered how such a simple known answer to this disease could exist without it being on the front cover of every newspaper,

The answer, I would learn, had deep political and financial roots. If simple apricot seeds were just one of the answers, as the orange was the answer to scurvy and died from scurvy, and the answer was simply vitamin C, found in an orange Just as the vitamin C in oranges was the Answer to scurvy and various B vitamins found in other simple foods had cured rickets and beri beri, apricot seeds could be the answer to so many prayers. And yet it was proving extremely difficult to get hold of.

I tried every pharmacy here in this country to locate vitamin $B_{17}$ made from apricot seeds, but it is not to be sold here. You can buy it in the States, but shipping it outside of the states is, for some unknown reason, forbidden.

I started to believe that what I had stumbled on made so much sense. I tried to find out why I could not get hold of simple $B_{17}$, made from apricot kernels. I continued to research, and I actually found out that, many years ago, people had eaten apricot seeds regularly in their diets, which cut the cases of cancer by half or more. Now it was time to find out why everybody wasn't aware of this and why I couldn't get a clear answer out of a doctor as to the benefits of laetrile, an injectable form of $B_{17}$.

After extensive research, I found that the one organization that most people put their trust in when it comes to food and medication safety, the FDA, had banned the sale of apricot seeds and refused to accept the truth about them, not allowing doctors to recommend this "home remedy". In fact, the FDA had jailed a man, Jason Vale, for selling apricot seeds after he was cured of his cancer—without the help of traditional medical remedies. This man was called crazy, even with proof that the seeds had cured his cancer.

Apricot seeds are naturally grown and are not money-maker's. Like Essiac's herbs, apricot seeds are naturally grown and proven to cure many cancers. But neither are money-makers. And just as I was learning how difficult it was to find apricot seeds, Rene Caisse had also run into profound difficulties trying to share her natural cure with the world. Imagine that—apricot pits or seeds from a God given fruit banned in the good ole USA.

Eventually, the FDA had no choice but to legalize the sale of apricot seeds, which are now available online at a fraction of the cost of most prescriptions. The judge ordered Vale's release and issued a statement to the FDA in which he noted that it appeared the only thing Vale was guilty of was trying to help people. However, this was after he had been locked up for *many* years.

Even so, the battle is far from over. To this day, doctors are not allowed to recommend apricot seeds for cancer treatment because, according to the FDA, laetrile is poisonous and has to be regulated.

At the time, my son was in the United States, and I was going to try to get hold of this product and have him bring some back with him. We would need enough that Perry could take 6 doses of 500 mg daily for as long as he had the cancer; he would cut the dosage once he was in the clear. And he would be!

I now had complete faith in what God had provided us humans as natural remedies for sickness. I had to, and I was more determined each day to share my experience with others. I would continue to share my testimony in my journal or on my blog, regardless of how many people chose to believe it. The battle wasn't over yet, but it would be.

I could only express the gratitude I felt from the bottom of my heart to the countless other people who had shared their testimonies— the stories of how they cured themselves of cancer by having enough self-motivation and discipline to try one of the oldest remedies out there. I was grateful for their courage and willingness to put their testimonies online in an effort to help others like me who only had the Internet as a source of comfort and knowledge. No one understands what you are going through unless they too have gone through it.

In the Bible, I'd read many things about God giving us all we need. In Genesis 1:29, he says, "I have given you every plant with seeds on the face of the earth and every tree that has fruit with seeds. This will be your food." This includes all grains, vegetables with seeds (beans, legumes, sesame, corn, and the like), nuts, and fruits. This was very interesting, considering everything I had read and seen in video testimonials, which told the stories of people curing their own diseases purely with nutrition and vitamins—natural therapies.

Doctors, on the other hand, stopped the pain with drugs—drugs that were manufactured and made for the profit of the pharmaceutical companies but left patients suffering from their side effects.

I soon found another cancer institute in America. The Bicher Cancer Institute (BCI) offered an alternative treatment for cancer

Hyperthermia, also known as thermal therapy or thermotherapy, application of localized heat to the tumour area at the temperature of 113°F or 42.5°C. Heat is known to be damaging to cancer cells, while safe to the normal tissue. The process is simple. Heat increases blood circulation; hence oxygenation of the cells, and oxygen is harmful to cancer cells. Studies show that hyperthermia is most effective in conjunction with other forms of cancer treatments, such as radiation therapy. Applying hyperthermia after the radiation treatment significantly improves the results. This approach, had been approved by the FDA in 1984, and prior to that, many studies were performed in the leading medical institutions around the world. Hyperthermia treatment has been used on different types of cancer, including skin, colon, neck, bladder, prostate, breast, base of tongue, throat, thyroid, and bone. BCI has been particularly successful in treating breast cancer, including inflammatory breast cancer (IBC), prostate, head and neck (throat, base of tongue, and tonsils), and skin cancers. The average success rate for early stages of breast cancer, including inflammatory breast cancer (IBC); prostate cancer; and head and neck cancers is about 80 per cent.

I contacted BCI and sent my husband's details there. We received a detailed statement of the costs of treatments needed and the length of time we would need. The institution recommended a twelve-week program, and the cost was around $55,000—not an option unless the insurance company would okay it. On with the next task—sending the details yet again to our insurer in the hopes that the company would help me look into a gentler form of treatment along these lines, to try to save my husband's bladder.

## 23 September: Two months after diagnosis

Five weeks after the second diagnosis, Perry and I were still researching. The more I'd looked into alternative herbal remedies, the stronger I felt that I didn't even want my husband to go to a cancer institutes at all. By now, I had learned that even immunotherapy included low doses of radiation. And I had come to firmly believe that we could cure Perry with nutrition and vitamin therapy, and I wanted to continue down this path.

Perry looked and felt so well. He was continuing to do his journeywork and to take the Essiac. We would have the vitamin $B_{17}$ that Wednesday, and he would start right away gradually building up his intake of the vitamin. I planned to document any progress.

## 24 September

We get another email informing us that the insurance company wouldn't cover the cost of thermal therapy as a treatment in America. The email explained that thermal therapy was still in the experimental stage and was not yet a proven cure. We were back to square one.

But I believed this was happening for a reason. My Intuition was telling us to go ahead with our nutritional and vitamin therapies to keep the cancer at bay. Perry was feeling well, and we would continue with the tests to see how he was medically.

We booked an appointment with a naturopathic doctor so that we could determine whether his body was in an alkaline or acidic state. We needed to keep his body's pH level alkaline. If his levels were acidic, that would indicate that he wasn't getting enough oxygen. I had learned that cancers thrive on this state.

Alkalizing his body did mean a radical change to his diet. Most importantly, he needed to add highly alkaline foods. Green vegetables are the most highly alkaline foods on the planet, and this would help his body counteract the acidic by-products of other foods with healthy alkaline by-products. He would also start drinking water with squeezed lemon juice a few times daily; although lemons are a known acidic fruit, once the fruit is in the body, it becomes alkaline, while fruits high in sugar are acid forming.

It was a lot to take in, but we were learning as we went. We wanted to do the best we could with what was available to us. The information was out there, and I was soaking it all up, though I had to go and seek it out first. Everything I needed to know was waiting for me, like a puzzle I was piecing together.

I urge everyone to read Knockout Interviews with Doctors Who Are Curing Cancer—And How to Prevent Getting It in the First Place by Suzanne Somers. Was a great help and Inspiration, to me.

As I was reading, I was filled with emotion. I wanted to read it to Perry, but I couldn't form the words; I was too choked up to read to him. Even though I had read and watched so many Testimonies from people whose message was the same as Somers's, I was shocked by what I read. This book, through many interviews with doctors, proved that cancer could be cured with the proper nutrition.

I received two letters back from doctors to whom I'd written—and I'd written to many, all over the world. Both gave me phone numbers and congratulated us on what we had done so far. Every day, I found something new to help me or someone came forward with a piece of interesting information. People who use alternative treatment approaches are extremely giving and helpful. They too have discovered invaluable information and want to spread the word. I had a full-time job, and I undertook it with all my passion—I would find a way to heal my beautiful man.

Most Oncologists say that the only three successful ways to cure cancer is chemo, surgery, and radiation, and two of those methods are poisonous to every cell in the body. Fear could have led us down the conventional path, and I now realized that is just what our doctors wanted—to catch us while the fear was ripe. Fear makes us believe we can do little on our own, making us trust the doctors who have studied so hard to become surgeons, oncologists, and the like. They didn't want to give us the time to make our own wise decisions based on thorough research into exactly what chemo entailed, what it did to the body.

If the doctors we'd seen had had their way, Perry would now be four weeks into chemotherapy and feeling unwell, off work, and very frightened. At the moment, he was happy, full of energy, and back to work, leaving all the researching to me. He could concentrate on something else, which was working for us both.

We now had a naturopathic doctor on board. She was very sympathetic to us both and said she didn't like cases like this but was willing to help us co-doctor him. She checked all his hormone levels to determine whether he had a vitamin deficiency. The consultation cost just over 100 pounds, and the blood tests cost the equivalent of 1,000 pounds. Three of the tests, which looked at Perry' oxygen levels, had to go to Germany, They were needed to see what vitamins and minerals his body was lacking in.

Our naturopath said we were doing the right thing with his diet and to carry on with the $B_{17}$, which cost 200 pounds for six weeks and which we were getting from the United States. She also gave us a whole list of vitamins and told Perry to take two tablespoons of apple cider vinegar in water every day to keep his body in an alkaline state. He'd had to drastically change his diet and had already cut out all pastries, cakes, chocolates, and snacks of every kind, except nuts and fruits. In addition, he'd cut out all rice, bread, potatoes, and alcohol.

All cow dairy products were out too. The food industry spends billions each year telling us milk does our bodies good, but really milk's acid content zaps our bones of acid neutralizers, which in turn, depletes our bone density. In addition, human beings stop developing lactase (the enzyme that breaks down milk sugar) between the ages of two and five. This means that, in adults who consume dairy products, undigested lactose ferments in the intestines, blocking the body from absorbing the good nutrients in foods and causing the immune system to stop working properly—in other words, diseases, like cancer.

Basically, Perry was now eating a plant-based diet, along with a little chicken and fish—poor thing. He'd already lost four kilograms, but he was looking good and feeling strong and well. Meanwhile, I was trying to educate myself on cooking different ways and on what to feed him to keep his strength and weight up once he got to his optimal weight (which would be after he'd lost possibly another four kilograms). I was trying not to let him lose it too quickly.

As you can imagine, being left to do all the research, cooking, shopping and trying to be sure I was feeding him the right things was very stressful. I sometimes become overwhelmed with this responsibility. At times, I had a few panic attacks in the grocery stores and health food shops as I read labels and determined what was or wasn't alkaline and so on.

We got the first batch of test results back from the naturopath, and almost all Perry's levels were okay. His vitamin D was almost completely depleted. I knew this was one thing to look out for in a cancer patient. Next, we would get the results of the tests that had been sent to Germany in two weeks.

## 27 September

I found yet another clinic in the United States that was doing clinical trials for the FDA to approve. The clinic had cured many cancers.

I wrote to the doctor there and found out that we would only need around three weeks there. Perry would be an outpatient for that period, after which he'd be sent home with lots of supplements. This treatment had something to do with the genes and peptides in patients with cancer. The researchers at the clinic had found a way to access the difference and reverse cancers in patients by adding what was missing in these patients who had no hope, even when the cancer had metastasized. It is hard to explain.

A Doctors assistant wrote back to me and told me the costs. Yet again, I sent this information off to our insurance company. I hadn't stopped researching from day one, and I would make sure my husband was well if it was the last thing I did.

Perry's state of mind was good, and he was doing everything that was required of him. He had initially been taking 500 mg of vitamin B$_{17}$ a day. Today, he doubled the dose to 1,000 mg. Each day, he will add 500 mg until he gets to around 4,000 a day. Using laetrile, the injectable form of vitamin B$_{17}$, would be better (if we could get it), as it is better tolerated at higher doses. With laetrile, he could get 6,000 mg into his system daily for twenty-one days before reducing to 1,000 mg daily. He would be rattling soon. He doesn't like taking tablets at the best of times, so I knew this must be really hard for him to do.

We had both been on a few walks on the beach as the sun went down, and it had been so relaxing for him. He told me he needed to do more of this—to just enjoy the beauty around us. He had also slowly started taking himself off to the gym for thirty minutes every few day; he was trying really hard to keep himself well and his spirits up.

One night, we watched a video together on Dr Burzynski, the doctor at the last clinic in the United States that I'd contacted. I was bought to tears. It was very informative. The Dr Burzynski movie full version, *A Cancer Cure*, is available on YouTube and about an hour and forty minutes long. It is well worth taking the time to look at; if nothing else, it will make you understand why we were choosing this clinic and doctor.

## 30 September

We got yet another email from our insurer. It stated:

> Kindly be informed that we have discussed the case. Personalized therapies are under trial and still not approved by FDA.

I could only hope we'd find a way. Though we'd saved a sizeable amount, I wasn't sure we had enough funds to cover all of the treatment. The cost could run far higher than we could possibly afford. What we needed now was a miracle.

## 1 October

We'd discussed over and over the benefits of going to the United States to the Burzynski clinic and had decided that we would go whether or not we got any help financially. If Perry was well, he could earn whatever we spent back. So we decided to go!

Our naturopath was being very supportive and urged us to go see Dr Burzynski if we could. She kindly asked me if I was okay, as she could see how stressed I'd become and used Perry's appointment to prescribe me some vitamins not available at normal health stores and only available through prescription from a trained certified naturopathic doctor. She also prescribed something to help with my hormones, without charging me for a consultation.

Perry had been a little down the last few days, but he'd had a lot on his plate at work at the moment. In addition, he really wanted to go to the United States to see what Dr Burzynski thought about helping him. While he didn't want to have another operation to find out if the cancer was still there, he felt guilty about the cost of going to the US clinic if what we were doing was keeping the cancer at bay anyway.

I had to keep letting him know that I supported him 100 per cent in whatever he wanted to do, that we would make up the money again, and that it meant nothing. If we'd saved for a rainy day, then it was pouring down at the moment, so we needed to use it.

I researched articles from reputable sites. We stayed away from the "junk sites", negative views on alternative medicine. And I searched for information specific to his diagnosis

Anyone who finds him or herself in this situation needs to have an advocate. It's hard to do it all yourself. Find someone you trust with the knowledge to do the research and ask for his or her help. Perry had me, and I got to work!

## Diet

I decided to make an effort to cut out all red meat and pork. Instead we chose fish and organic chicken where we could, and we swapped regular salt for sea salt, which isn't iodized.

We cut out all refined sugar, corn sugar, and high fructose corn syrup; instead we chose a natural sweetener, xylatol. Sugar to cancer is as gas is to fire! Natural or otherwise! Moderation is key. We never used artificial sweeteners, as none are safe.

We chose fresh over frozen and frozen over canned. We cut out flour and swapped white bread for Ezekial bread made from sprouted grains. Where possible Perry had 100 per cent wholemeal.

We swapped vegetable oil for cold pressed olive oil. For cooking, we used organic raw coconut oil or a pan that didn't require oil and had a lid with a seal so we could steam chicken and vegetables all at once. We swapped fried for grilled, baked, broiled, poached, or sautéed.

We swapped butter and margarine for a butter spread made with olive and nut oil. We swapped regular mayonnaise for one made with olive oil in moderation. We choose whole grain chips and crackers, baked when possible, and we swapped coffee for Sencha green tea.

We swapped dairy for almond milk or goat or camel milk and occasionally soymilk. We cut out all sugary drinks, including cokes, sweet tea, and fruit juices, which are high in sugar. We drank water with lemon juice added. We chose organic eggs and limited our intake to two or three per week if possible.

We choose turkey bacon over pork bacon and ground turkey over ground beef. We strictly cut out dairy products, eating small portions of goat cheese once in a great while. We steamed vegetables on the stove, not the microwave! We cooked and sliced our own meat for sandwiches, avoiding all processed meats.

## Vitamins and herbal remedies taken daily

Perry took two teaspoons of Essiac tincture in water three times daily; 3,000 mg of $B_{17}$ daily for twenty-eight days; 25 mg of DHEA, Dehydroepiandrosterone the most abundant hormone in the body. It is usually taken to enhance exercise performance or slow down the ageing process, prevent Alzheimer's, improve libido, fight fatigue, treat menopausal problems and build the immune system ; a high dosage of vitamin $D_3$ available only on prescription (20,000 mg daily for two weeks and then twice weekly); 30 mg of zinc daily; 30 mg of gut bug formula three times daily; and 1,000 mg of flax oil daily. In addition, he drank green powder detox drink twice daily for two weeks to flush out toxins and added high doses of vitamin C in powder form to his juices, which were mainly from vegetables.

## 3 October

The Burzynski Clinic sent us details of the next step. We needed to send off Perry's biopsy slides from his last biopsy. The great news was that we had them with us; I'd made sure we brought them back with us, which made me feel like I was in control of things. After the genetic testing results were back and the doctor had had time to review them, along with his other blood tests and records—a process that would take just over two weeks—we would be given an appointment time for a consultation. Things were moving forward!

All of life is a journey; what path we take, what we look back on, and what we look forward to is up to us. We determine our destination, what kind of road we take to get there, and how happy we are when we arrive.

## Saturday 6 October

The biopsy slides were on their way to Caris Laboratories in Arizona.

Scientific discoveries and technological breakthroughs had made it possible to examine cancers at a molecular level. Through advanced DNA, RNA, and protein analyses, the lab technicians could get a detailed molecular/genetic fingerprint of Perry's tumour to give to Dr Bursynski before we arrived for treatment. Then, based on these findings and Perry's current state of health, Dr Burzynski would decide on the best approach. The drugs were called targeted therapeutic agents. Some of these drugs might only be available through clinical trials, so only Dr Burzynski could decide whether Perry was a suitable candidate for them. All this would be done before we left for the clinic.

## Sunday, 7 October

Perry decided to make an appointment to see the urologist. He'd called the previous day, as we'd read about a blood test that looks for a tumour marker to determine whether the tumour is active. He asked if he'd already had this test, and the surgeon told him we haven't done it because they were going to remove the entire bladder.

At the appointment, Perry would have that test done, and we'd discuss with the surgeon the best way to check to see if the tumour has grown or stayed dormant and how often should he get checked.

We had been so busy looking for a cure that he'd forgotten to check to see if he was cured! He certainly looked well and felt well, and he had no pain whatsoever. He wasn't even feeling tired or depressed any more.

★   ★   ★

At the appointment, the urologist shared with us some information that he could never have shared unless we'd broached the subject ourselves. We informed him of what we were doing and told him we were looking into the Burzynski Clinic. He was already familiar with gene therapy and immunotherapy and started explaining why it wasn't allowed to be shared with patients.

We had a long conversation about alternative treatments, and he said he would do as we were doing if it were he in Perry's place, as he would go to God with his bladder intact. (Now that was coming from an urologist and surgeon who operates on bladders on a daily basis.)

We now knew we'd made the right choice. The surgeon told us of other alternative treatments that he knew worked. He explained that some were unethical, which was why the FDA wouldn't approve them. The worst of these he mentioned was a gene therapy in China that involved injecting cells from aborted human embryos. He said this could lead to women being paid to get pregnant to abort the embryo. Shocking but true.

I thought that this doctor could be on our side now, and he ordered all the tests he could to check on Perry. I told him all the things we were doing and said he could be cured now. But how, I asked, do we find out?

He explained that he could check Perry's cells in urine and blood tests and then perform another cystoscopy.

We were now waiting for approval from the insurance company to do the tests, along with another MRI. Then we could get on with it.

We returned home from the appointment feeling a lot happier; we could at least see that things hadn't gotten any worse and we were on the right track. I felt that the results of today's efforts were good.

## Wednesday, 10 October

I received two really nice and very encouraging messages from friends yesterday. Both told me they felt privileged to know me. I felt so loved and worthwhile. One of these friends had read my journal, and one hadn't. But both knew what I was undertaking—all my research and everything else I was involved with in my attempt to do whatever I could to be there 100 per cent for my husband. I got to think how hard it must be for friends, not knowing what to say or do to help. So I decided I would write a little of what was happening to me at this time:

> Sometimes I do feel like I am drowning in all this responsibility. Every step is a journey, and this is a serious journey. But I have to remember that Perry is also still a normally functioning person at home and at work. It's hard for people to understand how we live in both worlds at the same time, but we have to. Cancer not only attacks the body; it also takes its emotional and financial toll and that is a lot to deal with. Perry may look well enough on the outside, but still he is suffering, and sometimes I wish his friends would come around and take him out. My friends have been great. I have been treated to a spa day and lunches, and it is so nice to know my close friends

are trying in their own way to help us out, not just because they care but also because they know we are trying to go to this clinic and need all the money we can for it.

I wish people could understand how emotionally vulnerable we are, as he has not long been diagnosed and we have rejected all normal treatments. It is still a very scary predicament to be in. I mostly appreciate closeness, warmth, encouragement, and companionship. I do not need sympathy. I don't appreciate it when friends say, "Hush, everything is okay. You will be just fine. You don't have anything to worry about." I think it's important to remain positive and optimistic, but it's equally important to be realistic. I also do not appreciate people who tell me stories of other people who died of cancer. That is just not helpful. Perry is not his diagnosis and does not want to tell everyone he hasn't seen for a long time either.

I also need friends and family to understand that, when I forget what you just told me, I'm not demented or depressed or not paying attention. Stress messes with my short-term memory. I know this is happening more to him, but we are in this together and I am living it too as if it were me. The worst part is the fear of waiting for his test results. What a nervous wreck he has become before his MRI, which in turn makes me feel nervous as we wait for his appointment and medical tests he needs to see if what we are doing is working. And how I worry about every ache and pain that he has—does this mean he is getting worse? Just remember, if you don't know what to say or do, showing up, lending an ear, and remaining positive no matter what will mean the world.

We are still waiting to hear today when his MRI scan will be, and he is so nervous. But I feel this needs to be done before we take the next step in our Journey and go to the Burzynski Clinic, this MRI could mean what we have done so far has cured him and I am feeling very positive so actually quite excited to know but I realize my husband is against having it done as he doesn't want bad news.

## Friday, 12 October

Perry was now jogging in the park with me a few mornings a week. He is getting fitter and looks healthy and strong. He feels full of energy and is now on a full dosage of the vitamin $B_{17}$. He had decided to take the maximum dosage, 4,000 mg daily for twenty-one days and 1,000 mg after this period.

We were managing his food much better now, and his weight loss had almost stopped, which we were pleased about. He was getting lots of nutrition from juicing, as well as from the food he was eating. He still had five more days of detoxing with his green juices twice daily. Hopefully, after that, the nutrition with all the fruit and vegetable juices would be enough to maintain his immune system and build it up to the point that it would be doing its job of fighting the cancer cells itself. We now had to wait until Tuesday for his blood test and MRI scan.

## Monday, 15 October

It was one more day before Perry's MRI, and he was getting really anxious. His nervousness was obvious. I was trying to think positively;

at the moment I was quite excited to find out whether what we had done so far had worked for him. He certainly looked like it was working, and he had so much energy now. He even bought some new jogging shoes today, went out especially to buy them.

I received the loveliest email from my mother, giving me praise and encouragement for what I was doing. It was just what I needed to know. I had my family behind me, and for them to know how much all of this meant to me was especially meaningful.

# CHAPTER 4

## COPING WITH DISAPPOINTMENT

**Wednesday, 17 October**

Today was a day of great disappointed. We get the MRI results, and right before the appointment, the doctor Reschedules for Sunday, as the blood and urine cytology needed to be there so we'd have the whole picture. It would be a few more days before those results came back now. We could do nothing but wait until Sunday evening.

**Saturday, October 20**

As I struggled to get on with my day, I felt increasing pressure. What if Perry wasn't cured? What if I was just hoping he was better? Then I was reminded to take each day one step at a time and try as much as possible to stay in the present. Dwelling on something would never change the outcome, and worrying about the future with all its what ifs was just a waste of energy.

So I chose to have a wonderful day, whatever happened.

A beautiful day starts with a beautiful mind-set, where we take a moment to appreciate the little things and count our blessings, rather than focus on our problems we were saving energy, and making space for gratitude.

So this morning I decided to appreciate the opportunity to change what I could, starting with myself, and a smile on my face.

## Sunday, 2 October

Today could not come quickly enough. All day I was on edge, just waiting for our appointment time.

I was ecstatic when we finally learned that his tumour marker had come back negative, which didn't mean he was in the clear but simply that nothing was showing any progression and that at least the cancer cells hadn't spread or metastasized to other organs. The doctor kept reminding us that he could only tell us scientifically whether something was working.

I kept asking him to just tell us Perry wasn't getting any worse and that we could proceed with what we were doing.

He took us to see the radiologist who'd performed the last MRI. He showed us a slight thickening on the bladder wall, which wasn't normal. Yet neither he nor the urologist could say it was a cancerous growth, scar tissue, or a mass. We compared the scan to the previous one, and it clearly showed a reduction on the thickest part of the bladder wall from 14mm to 8mm, a difference in just 8 weeks The Doctor had no scientific evidence as to how this had happened, as this was not even the location from where the tumour was taken.

This alone made us so happy. We were on the right track, and at the moment, we didn't have to move on to plan B.

The doctor was concerned that Perry had some microscopic blood in his urine, which indicated an infection, along with the thickening on the bladder wall. He would have presumed the latter was owing to a growth, but after the cytology came back indefinite for malignancy present, he was left unsure.

We spoke about what we'd been doing, and the doctor commented on how well Perry was looking. His blood pressure had returned to normal, and he was healthy in every other aspect. I mentioned that he was jogging now, and he told us this could be the reason for the infection and blood in the urine. So he prescribed an antibiotic that Perry was to take for five days and asked us to return in a week for follow-up urine cytology's to rule out a growth as the reason for blood in the urine. In addition, he suggested that Perry have another cystectomy (biopsy) in about four to six weeks to test what cells were still in the thickening of the wall.

Other than that he couldn't comment on the treatments we were doing. But he had told us Perry hadn't gotten any worse and commented on how healthy and how much younger Perry was looking. We were excited and yet still worried, although it had relieved a lot of pressure to move onto our next step.

I was very glad we had such an understanding urologist now. He clearly liked us and was helping us do as many tests as were available to see that Perry hadn't gotten any worse. Meanwhile, we could continue along the path we had chosen.

We were doing so many things that we didn't have a clue which one was working. So we would just continue them all, except for the jogging. We would have to limit our exercise to walking for a while.

I was so happy tonight.

## 23 October

For some reason, I wanted to muse over some of the treatments we were doing. I started with the Essiac tincture, which Perry had now been taking continuously for six weeks. I again researched how the combination of herbs worked on cancer and came across something that would explain the thickening found on the wall of Perry's bladder. The Sovereign's Health Freedom Network, in an article on its website called "How does Essiac tea work on cancer and are there any side effects?" reported:

Most importantly . . . it was discovered that one of the most dramatic effects of taking this remedy was its affinity for drawing all the cancer cells which had spread back to the original site at which point the tumour would first harden, then later it would soften, until it vanished altogether or more realistically, the tumour would decrease in size to where it could then be surgically removed with minimal complications.

In certain cases and at certain stages of the disease, the cancer would act as if it were "coming to a head", similar to an abscess. It would then break down and slough away.

If this had happened with the cancer in Perry's bladder, then this would account for the thickening seen on his latest MRI scan. All we could do was wait for another six weeks to pass to get yet another MRI to compare it to. Also by this time, he would have taken the full dosage of $B_{17}$ and would be back down to the dosage recommended for preventative care. This too should have a profound effect on the cancer. He would take another urine sample to make sure the infection was gone and then make the appointment for the next MRI in four to six weeks.

## 29 October

I had been thinking a lot lately about what would have happened if we had not returned home and taken the time to consider our options. Once you have been given the diagnosis, your mind is in a whirl, you can't think straight, and you're scared out of your wits. The cancer industry has you right where it wants you. It is ingrained in everyone that, if you have cancer, you are more than likely going to die. Weighed down by the feelings that come with that idea, you are in no condition to investigate alternatives.

If, by sharing my journal, I can give someone else the strength to gather their thoughts enough to start investigating what cancer really is and how it should be treated, I will have done what I set out to do. Your doctors know that you would run from them and their poisons, if you fully understood. That's why the pressure on you is so intense.

Does a person get cancer because he is suffering from a deficiency of surgery, radiation, chemotherapy, and drugs? Once you realize that the answer to this question is obviously no, you will see that traditional "standard of care" treatments, even if administered at state-of-the art cancer clinics, have no cure to offer you. You don't need to rush to sign up for those treatments. You really can afford to take the time to relax and regain your composure and then decide on a rational approach based on alternatives that do offer you the potential for a complete cure. Whether you have a lot of money or not, and even if you have no health insurance, you really can make a complete recovery from cancer.

At only ten weeks post diagnosis, Perry was doing great. This was why I would continue to keep my journal—in the hope that, one day, someone would read it and take a little hope and guidance from what I had learned and what Perry had put into practice.

Either way, you will discover that you are always in control of your body. You may either use your energy for nourishing and healing the body or waste it on fighting a battle against a disease that medical theory believes is out to kill you. The choice is ultimately yours, but to realize you do have a choice is a wonderful awakening. Bottom line, the main issue in question is not whether you have cancer but how you perceive it and what you are going to do about it. If you look at it as your body's way of forcing you to alter the way you see and treat yourself, including your physical body. You may either make out cancer to be something dreadful that leaves you victimized and powerless or see it as an opportunity to stand up for yourself and your values and regain some self-respect.

## 5 November

We finally got the results of the urine analysis back, and it showed no infection and no blood in the urine, which meant it must have been the jogging causing the blood. All we could do now was carry on with our alternative medicines and de-stress tactics until Perry's next MRI in around four weeks. By then he would have been taking a full dosage of $B_{17}$, so we might see a better result. But we know you can't rush these things.

Perry left for the United States on business. It was the first time he'd been away from me since his diagnosis, so it was hard for me not to worry. He was clued up on what he could and could not eat, so if he kept to his diet and took his vitamins and Essiac, there should be no problems.

He had no stress, no pain, no urgency to urinate, no microscopic blood, no frequency, no burning, no incontinence, no leaking, and no symptoms. Was he cured? He was living with it was all we could say at the moment. He felt like the only problem he had was coping with his diet—not a bad thing, considering he should now be without his bladder and trying to recover.

## Making decisions together

I guess some people don't want a lot of information because they aren't sure they can handle what the possibilities are. But I don't think you can really make a good decision without knowing everything. We had to ask a lot of questions, though, because we didn't know all our options.

Now we were armed with the knowledge and a true belief that our thoughts were mainly responsible for whether we would heal. And it was equally as important to remain stress free and happy, as it was to keep your body fuelled with energy, giving it raw and as natural as possible foods.

Dr Leonard Coldwell's book, *The Only Answer to Cancer*, was a great inspiration to me when it came to changing both my husband's and my own diet. He was motivated, like I'd been, by his family members and loved ones contracting cancer. And he'd seen first-hand how chemo and radiation did nothing but cause their deaths.

Coldwell has spent his life's work trying to get the word across that cancer can be cured, naturally by our own healthy cells, along with a healthy mind, body, and spirit. I urge everyone to read his book and look at some interviews that are out on the Internet about him and what he has done to cure thousands of patients from cancer.

Every day, I thanked God that we'd stayed away from the chemo and radiation and had opted; instead to first try all these other natural remedies, as well as reducing Perry's stress levels. To do that, he slowed down his workload and stopped all his travel for a while, as well as late-night conference calls. We went for walks on the beach and walked and exercised outdoors to get fresh air in his lungs and sunlight on his skin. We also became quite selfish and did what Perry wanted to do, instead of what he felt he should do. We booked a cruise so that we could totally relax over Christmas instead of travelling to England and staying with relatives the entire time. Our family are all well meaning, but they made Perry feel like he needed looking after (like he was really sick). We decided it would be better to just go relax where no one would feel sorry for him or give him unwanted advice.

Of course, we did need to see our family, and our sons needed to see their father. But we decided we could do that for a short period of time that would allow us to simply enjoy the time with our grandchildren and then go on to a cruise to relax on our own.

Today, my husband was to return from his business trip. I'd been so worried that he'd have gotten stressed while he was there. He said he was fine, just stressed about what was available to eat and the lack of fresh juices. I'd been shopping to make sure I could feed him well today, stocking up on everything that he likes. I felt like I'd been making him eat only certain things, and I felt sorry that I couldn't be there to go look for things for him while he was working.

He sent me a photo of him with a very good friend who'd travelled to where Perry was staying to see him after nearly twelve years of not seeing each other. The photograph first made me smile, but then I saw my husband in a different light. He looked so much smaller in frame, and his skin looked different. His washed-out appearance could have been a result of the flash, but I was concerned. Perry looked so tired.

I reflected that his weariness could also be due to the nine-hour time difference, which led me to wonder if he was ready to make these long-haul flights. He was trying to get his immune system in peak condition. How did these flights affect your system? I needed to research this too.

I considered that he had to wake at four in the morning and drive for three hours to the airport. That was followed by a two-hour wait and a fourteen-hour flight. All of that would be hard for the fittest person to endure.

I was so glad he had me to take care of him while he was home. What would he do if he were alone on this journey?

## 12 November

The doctor called and told Perry he had positive cells in his urine, which meant microscopic blood again. He was due to go on another business trip, which he couldn't get out of, and decided to take another week-long course of antibiotics with him and then go to see the doctor In a week to take another sample.

I was very worried. I wanted to know what was causing this. Previously, we'd been told it could be the jogging, so we'd stopped that. Now we just don't know what to think.

I didn't want him to have another biopsy, as I'd read that many cancers metastasized because of the biopsy—when tumours were cut into they could release a protein that could spread the cancer cells. It was all getting too much for me to deal with, especially while he was traveling and I couldn't take care of him.

All I could do now was hope these antibiotics worked and that he would manage to get plenty of rest while he was away. He had no visual blood in the urine and no pain and said he felt well and full of energy. He certainly looked well. Maybe I was worrying unjustly.

If we were to ask most doctors whether cancer could be cured, they would say they could do a lot of things to slow it down but, to be honest, until they addressed the root cause, the cancer would continue to thrive and grow back elsewhere in the body, Perry's immune system was in peak condition now, and it showed in his outlook and temperament. The nagging backache that had once plagued him just twenty weeks earlier had disappeared. He didn't fall asleep in the evening while watching TV. He woke without an alarm and jumped out of bed full of energy. He was able to do these long-haul flights and conduct stressful meetings with a clear head—and all because of his diet and vitamin therapy, which was building not only his immune system but also his hormone balance as well. This kept his moods level. In addition, blood pressure problems or cholesterol issues no longer troubled him, and all we are doing seemed to have corrected all of his other niggling little health problems, along with the feeling of lethargy and depression. He had a very high level of energy, and an immense feeling of wellness had come about him.

## 18 November

Perry had another appointment with the urologist. He had been quite supportive and interested in what we were doing, but after the urine cytology came back positive for cancer cells and microscopic blood, he now told us he wanted to do another biopsy. We both had a long chat with him again, explaining that we didn't want another surgery or more anaesthesia, as this would deplete his immune system after we had built it up to peak condition. We had to believe in what we were doing. We had come this far, and we'd gotten a great result with the last MRI.

We made a deal with him. We would have another MRI first, and then it showed anything we should worry about, we would go ahead with his wishes. Perry wanted to wait until after Christmas for the next MRI. We had all agreed on this plan around the beginning of January.

I had been continuing to research alternative treatments. I think maybe what the doctor told us had knocked my confidence a little. I was consumed by two thoughts—the conviction that what we were doing was working and the realization that perhaps we needed to pay more attention to the seriousness of this illness. I could see Perry was well at the moment, but this last visit had definitely upset me, as the doctor had stressed again that he was just worried for Perry, and although he admired what we were trying to do, he had to tell us that the best chance of recovery was to remove his bladder completely.

I already knew what all the doctors were saying, but I'd been hoping that this one would just keep helping us to make sure Perry wasn't getting any worse, allowing us to keep the tumour under control and, therefore, keep his bladder. Sadly, this was beyond his capability. So I soon set to work yet again. Every spare minute I had was devoted to research.

# CHAPTER 5

## DIFFICULT DECISIONS

I came upon an amazing video interview about cannabis oil. It completely blew my mind. I had watched countless videos and read so many testimonials about it by this point. I'd even mentioned the oil's healing potential to the doctor. He'd laughed and said cannabis oil was very potent and illegal and warned us not to bring it into the Middle East. He didn't say that I was talking rubbish or that it wouldn't work; he simply warned me about its illegality.

We both made a life-changing decision we told the urologist we didn't want the chemo and that the treatment we were adopting was our opportunity for us to heal my husband holistically. He wasn't happy but gave us an appointment for the MRI in January 2013, to satisfy himself whether or not the tumour had grown or spread.

I met some interesting people on Facebook who had a lot to say about cannabis oil curing cancer. I did all the research I could and only came up with positive things about the plant. The testimonials of people who had been cured were incredible. I can't mention names, but I wrote on the wall of one of the groups that is fighting to legalize cannabis, asking if anyone knew where I could get my hands on some cannabis oil. I already knew about the oil's benefits

I managed to connect with some people who were taking the legal issue to Courts within the Uk and America; these people could put me in contact with others who were growing the herb to help heal people with cancer. If I could get hold of it, I estimated the cost to be around 2,000 English pounds.

Cannabis oil is very strong and the idea is to build up the daily dose over time. One dose is a drop on your finger about the size of a grain of rice.

Loads of sites give information about cannabis oil. One of the best is Phoenix Tears, located at http://phoenixtears.ca/make-the-medicine.

I felt strong, brave, and invincible. I would do anything in my power to get this medicine for my husband. I was extremely tired by this point as my research started yet again. My plan was now to source this medicine and bring it here where he could take it daily.

What I'd come to realize through this experience is that we alone are responsible for our health, and it's up to ourselves to heal our own bodies. No doctor can do that. In fact, no doctor will help you take the alternative route to healing. Most of all, no one knows what's best for us except us. The doctor had to tell us what he knew, and all he knew was about chemo, radiation, and surgery. He had no knowledge of how alternative medicine worked. I had to trust my instincts but remain grounded; I had to understand that if Perry started showing any signs that the route we had taken wasn't working, then we should listen to the doctor. I didn't want to say goodbye to my husband at any cost.

If this story encourages someone in a similar situation to do the same, then my reason for writing this has been achieved! I'd spent many months now researching every aspect of cancer and the holistic healing modalities to cure it or at least put up a bigger fight against it, which is better than what chemo can do for you. If this story helps others to make the same move, then all this stress and hard work will have paid off.

Lastly, I have to say that Perry's cancer diagnosis was a true blessing. It facilitated a change within me on every level—emotionally, physically, mentally, and spiritually. It formed an unbreakable bond of love and support between my husband and me. I'd become brave and confident in my own power, and this was truly the biggest blessing. I really want to help inspire others to do the same.

## 21 November

The doctor texted a message that Perry's urine cytology had come back with no microscopic blood, no cancer cells, and no infection. This was great news for us, as perhaps the presence of blood had been worrying the doctor. That was why he'd told us Perry would have the best chance if he removed his bladder. He'd felt that the return of the blood in the urine was a sign that the cancer had started to metastasize.

## 23 November

I'd had three days of chronic headaches. I supposed I wasn't as brave as I thought I was.

I'd also managed to source three places to get the cannabis oil. Following through on any of them would be risky, as the oil was illegal in England and more so here in the Middle East.

One of the places I'd sourced was a medical centre in Holland. Getting the oil through this centre would require Perry having an appointment with a certified doctor to get a prescription to buy the oil. The product would at least come from a proper medical laboratory, so we would know it was the correct strength. But we also knew Perry would need a three-month supply, which would cost around 2000 pounds

I'd done quite a lot of work to get this information, but these headaches were there for a reason. Possibly, they were warning me to think very carefully before going ahead with this route. I was in tune with my intuition, and I knew instinctively that this wasn't the way at the moment.

Perry and I both agreed that what we were already doing was clearly working, so there was no need to go this step further and get the oil just yet. But it was good to know it was out there should there come a time when we absolutely needed the oil If we found we needed to take the treatment one step further, with a plant extract, even if it was an illegal one, we would. I knew for fact cannabis oil stopped many kinds of pain. I knew that doctors gave it to cancer patients. The problem lay with the government, as it can't figure out how to get its "share" from anyone who uses it.

I was inspired and motivated. I felt strong and empowered again about our lifestyle decisions. Not enough people are aware of what is possible just by giving our body what it needs. The solutions to many of our health issues are so simple and so natural! Nourish your body, and your body will fix itself.

## 24 November

I received an email from our naturopathic doctor sending me an article about using baking soda in water twice a day to raise the alkalinity of the body's pH levels. Perry's diet was already raising the alkalinity slightly, but our naturopath explained that it needed to be higher to kill cancer cells. I went to work once again.

There is much evidence that most people over the age of fifty are suffering from acid overload. When our body's pH is too acidic, we are vulnerable to all kinds of diseases. Bacteria, mould, yeast and fungi thrive in an acidic environment.

I had done a great deal of research on alkalizing the body through diet, and this was really hard to achieve. PH levels within the human body are important; the comprehensive approach to raising the body PH levels is by, first taking a test to check if increasing pH levels is needed for you. Then eat foods that are high in alkaline these include most fruits and vegetables like Broccoli, cabbage, asparagus which are high in alkaline and avoid high acidity foods like soda, red meats coffee among many other's Consuming raw foods was the primary way to raise pH levels, and at 8.5, cancer couldn't survive. A normal rate would be around 6.5 anything below this and you probably have cancer. It was almost impossible to achieve an elevated alkalinity with diet alone. But now I saw a speedy way to do it—drinking bicarbonate of soda in water. If it worked, I would document the changes.

Using special strips bought at the pharmacy, you can test your urine in the morning to check your body's pH level Perry had had a healthy diet for around three months now. He had also quit smoking And yet, when we tested his urine, his pH balance was at a 6—in the normal range. For urine pH a 7 or higher is alkaline.

## 29 December

It was now 29 December. Christmas had come and gone, and we are anxious to get Perry's MRI sorted. Today, we scheduled an appointment. The doctor would call us with a date as soon as we got the okay from the insurance company.

Perry's weight had plateaued now at around ninety kilograms, which meant he'd lost a total of seven kilograms and then maintained his weight now for over three weeks. His appetite was good, and it was probably down to the hormone DHEA, which the naturopath had prescribed.

Perry continued to take all his alternative medications. He was getting enough sleep, and he wasn't stressed, or not visibly anyway! He looked and felt really well. Now all we needed was confirmation from the MRI that what we were doing was continuing to serve him well.

At this point, his pH level was between 7 and 8, and he'd only been taking a half teaspoon of bicarbonate in water each day to help keep his levels up and to ensure that his pH levels wouldn't slip into an acidic state.

A few people had asked to see my journal lately, as friends and family members had found out that their loved ones had been diagnosed. Their desire to share my journal made me feel very proud. All the research I'd done and the documentation of our progress could benefit someone else. I could, perhaps, help others and they could get tips about where to research things and wouldn't have to spend so long getting the answers they needed to inform themselves.

I was so looking forward to the impending MRI. (Was that normal?) I was amazed by what was happening and what I'd learned, and I wondered why *cancer* was such a dreaded word if all you had to do was give your body the right tools to heal itself.

A combination of a raw food diet and herbal remedies could shrink tumours and help reverse cancer, all while improving the quality of life for cancer survivors. Moreover this combination could help bring down the number of people who were diagnosed every year.

I'd become a strong advocate of using herbal medicine and eating a diet free of processed foods. Had I not educated myself about cancer and its causes when we discovered that my husband had bladder cancer, I may have made the grave mistake of being overcome with fear and, thus, pushing him towards a medical doctor to get mutilated in surgery, radiated to death, or poisoned to death with chemotherapy treatments.

I hope that, one-day, our story will help others learn to adopt an alternative approach to healing.

Taking full control and responsibility of our own individual health is one of the most revolutionary non-violent actions we can make. This is especially important in a time when government officials are trying to pigeonhole us into a health care system that railroads us straight into the grasps of medical and pharmaceutical industries, whose monetary greed causes them to embrace death and disease, rather than life and good health.

## 2 January

I was back on track with all my research. We needed to get this MRI over with; from its results, we would draw some encouragement to carry on and stay the course, show the world that alternative treatment works, and give others some hope and encouragement.

Perry managed to get through Christmas eating healthy and keeping his pH levels above 7, which was quite an achievement, as he drank red wine and a little whiskey and had a lot of extra food. As for the food, I cooked it especially for him with organic coconut oils instead of vegetable or olive oil. Coconut oil is really much tastier anyway. In fact, the entire family and all our guests ate oven roasted veg in extra virgin organic coconut oil and all remarked how much tastier the veg was. I even made Perry's favourite fried dumplings and jerk chicken in the oil.

I decided to try and eat just like he was. He had maintained his weight goal. As I didn't want to lose lots of weight, I'd only cut out some foods. But seeing how much healthier Perry was and how much energy he had, I made my New Year's resolution to feed myself the same way I fed my husband. The hardest things for me to cut out would be sugar and dairy, but I was going to give it a go.

The only way for us all to get and stay healthy is to take charge, take responsibility, and take control of our own lives and health. We must get educated; use common sense; and listen to our instincts—intuition is there for a reason—and then apply what we learn. Ask yourself, "What is it that made me sick?" or "What could have been the reason or one of the reasons for me getting sick?"

One main cause of cancer is stress. Scientific studies have proven that 86 percent of all illnesses and doctor visits are stress-related. Illness is lack of energy. The main cause of lack of energy is mental and emotional stress.

We were all born with cancer, yet our bodies simply eliminated all the danger and debris, the toxins and acidosis in our body so that the cancer couldn't grow or take over. The only way that process is stopped is when our immune system gets compromised and no longer has the strength to eliminate the accumulation and multiplication of cancerous cells.

The only way to get and stay healthy is to get our energy level back up to where it needs to be for the healing process. Therefore, we first need to eliminate the physical foundation for cancer, acidosis and toxaemia.

The fastest way of this is to use a massive cleansing system like the one our naturopath prescribed—green powder detox cleansing powder, along with Essiac tincture or capsules. In addition, avoid sugar or artificial sweeteners and start juicing; drink a third each of apple, carrot, and celery juice every morning. In fact, juice as much as you can each day and add lots of greens, like spinach and parsley, for the chlorophyll present in it. (This gives the body oxygen.)

Never drink cows' milk (check out www.notmilk.com). Cut out red meat.

Max Plank and Otto Warburg received a Nobel Prize in medicine for proving that cancer couldn't exist in an oxygen-rich alkaline environment. If you were to do all of the above, you'd be detoxified, your body's pH levels would be alkaline, and you'd have enriched your body with oxygen. That means you'd have eliminated the physical cause and the foundation for cancer in your body.

The problem was that people believed the media and didn't believe that cancer could be cured. It was hard to get people to understand that the media's goal wasn't to inform but to control. It wasn't that I thought I was smarter than Perry's doctors. It was simply that I cared more about him than anyone else did.

The problem with building the immune system was that it was a slow process. My husband was lucky; he had the time and the energy to rebuild it. Many cancer patients who'd sought out natural cancer treatments had been sent home to die and the time they had left to live wasn't long enough to rebuild their immune system after it had been damaged by chemotherapy. But we were lucky; we had listened to our instincts before resorting to chemotherapy, radiotherapy and surgery. In fact, we would never have had the second biopsy done if we'd known then what we knew now—that anaesthetic and surgery depletes the immune system further.

## 5 January

Perry had his MRI today. Our Radiologist and his team spent three whole hours looking for cancer. They even used contrast dye after the plain one. They couldn't find anything. But they knew Perry hadn't undergone chemo or radiation, so they wondered where the cancer had gone and kept looking.

The radiologist weren't allowed to tell us much, but they did say they couldn't see anything serious except for an irregularity in the ureter. They assured us, however, that this was nothing to worry about and that we could come back tomorrow to speak with both the urologist and the radiologist. The head of the radiology department was to be there too and we were to bring Perry's previous MRI results—from the one he'd had in England, as well as from the first MRI in July when he was diagnosed, and the one he'd here nine weeks ago.

I wasn't too worried about the irregularity they'd found, as the surgeon in England had told us Perry had an out-pouching in his bladder that he'd been born with. (The medical term for this type of hollow or fluid-filled structure was diverticulum.) This radiologist didn't know this. Still, I wouldn't be sleeping much tonight.

## Sunday, 6 January

I realized I should, perhaps, wait a while before writing, as I was a little upset and not sure what to think. All the excitement of yesterday had been washed away with our appointment today, and I needed time to sit down and digest it all.

It wasn't all doom and gloom, and a lot of positives had come out of the appointment. But we were definitely not yet in the all-clear department. I felt as if we'd both taken a knock, and it would take some time for us to decide what our next move should be. I always wrote better when I didn't have too much time to think about what to write. It helped me figure things out. It was difficult for me to talk at the moment but needed to share, which was why I was writing.

It had been a long wait while the three doctors discussed all the different MRIs Perry had had before inviting us in for a chat. The urologist had always maintained that Perry needed to have his bladder removed, as his cancer was invasive, which meant it was into the muscle wall. But when he'd seen nine weeks ago that the cancer had regressed, he hadn't known what to make of it. He'd kept insisting we do another biopsy, as there was still some thickening on the bladder wall. We'd made a deal to wait until after Christmas for another MRI, and then, if the scan showed that the cancer had progressed, we would decide to have a cystectomy and biopsy.

Yesterday's MRI results had shown no cancer in the bladder. The radiologist had said there was no change. I too could see that his bladder was clear. I had watched each stage and knew what to look for now.

The radiologist said everything looked fine in the bladder, but he saw a little problem in the ureter. Perry had always thought that the original tumour was in the bladder and slightly up the ureter on the right side. The two urologist specialists disagreed on this point. The one in England said the tumour had not gone into the ureter, and this one here thought it had initially.

As the urologist here could plainly see, the cancer in the bladder had not progressed as of now, and the radiologist told us there was no change from the results of the MRI Perry had had nine weeks ago. (In my mind, no progression was excellent news.) The Urologist knew he had no chance of persuading us to have the cystectomy (another biopsy) and an exploratory under anaesthetic on the original site. Now he insisted that he needed to do a biopsy and exploratory examination of the ureter.

We were now left with a decision—whether or not to go ahead with the biopsy. We had to decide whether this doctor was just trying to get the money the insurance would pay for the hospital here while putting my husband's immune system in jeopardy once again.

This was a very difficult decision. We decided once again what to believe. Given that the cancer in the bladder had not progressed, had not metastasized to other organs, and had not reached any lymph nodes, should we trust that the doctor was right about what was causing a kink in perry's ureter? Or should we trust that, with all we were doing, the cancer would regress if we gave it a little more time.

I decided to look into how much this biopsy would affect his immune system and weigh up the pros and cons of having it done.

## 7 January

I was feeling a little more positive. It had been hard for me to even think straight yesterday, never mind have a conversation with anyone. I was happy that I'd written it all down and sent emails out instead of talking to anyone. That way, I just listened to my inner voice and not what our family thought we should do out of fear. I had gotten very good at closing myself off to the outside influence of family and friends who hadn't done the research I had. I felt increasingly alone.

I could only imagine Perry's reaction to be the same. We couldn't even talk to each other. It was as if we were both numb and needed time to contemplate and digest it all before deciding what to do.

Now, after giving each other space, we both came to the same conclusion alone in the night. I woke at three and was downstairs until five. Perry got out of bed at five. Neither of us spoke about the decision we'd been contemplating until lunchtime today. When

Perry came home from work, I cooked his lunch and called him, asking that he come home so we could talk. I told him my thoughts, and he said he'd had the same thoughts and had been thinking this all night.

We both could see clearly what we needed to do. First, we needed to change doctors. We needed to find someone who wasn't so negative towards alternative therapies and get a second opinion about the MRI scans. I'd already written to our naturopath and told her everything; in the hope she would know of another doctor she could ask to look at his MRI and his urine cytology.

Things just didn't add up to me. Yesterday, our doctor had told us Perry's last urine cytology had shown cancer cells and blood, and I knew his last cytology had come back clear. Our doctor was trying to use the previous test results to persuade us that it was highly likely Perry had a malignancy. Then when I'd ended up raising my voice; that his last cytology had come back negative for blood, cancer cells and bacteria, he'd said I was wrong. I'd told him he had lots of patients and had been for a Christmas break, and I had just one husband whom I was taking care of! I knew what his last results had told us word for word.

When we returned home, he'd sent an email:

This is what I mean!!

He'd attached the report from October, which had shown blood and bacteria in Perry's urine, and not the last one he'd done in November.

I knew then that we had to change doctors. The urologist didn't realize we had a hard copy of all of Perry's records. The doctor had initially just texted the results to my phone, but I'd insisted we go to the hospital and get a copy of the results, as the urologist had gone on vacation the nursing staff had just printed it out for us without question, and this report included the negative result, which stated "no need for follow up".

I'd slept on it, and now I was back on track looking for another doctor.

Our naturopath sent me a lovely email. She expressed that she felt we were doing the right thing in wanting a second opinion and recommended a very good radiologist at her clinic. She wanted this doctor to have a look at all of the MRI results, and she also wanted to do some blood work, which would show any reasons for concern.

We set the appointment for Thursday, 10 January, in two days' time. Then, depending on their findings, we would find another urologist to do a biopsy.

## 9 January

When something bad happens, we can either let it define us, let it destroy us, or let it strengthen us. The choice is ours. We are still a work in progress, which means we will get to where we want to be a little at a time. No matter how many times I'd broken down, there was always a voice inside me that said, "No, you're not done yet! Get back up!" And I did.

It was certainly hard at the moment not to slip into feeling sorry for myself. I was trying so hard not to, but the tears I held onto were making it difficult to hide my sorrow. Friends and family were noticing that I was consumed by it all. I'd lost a few friends already, but it has been good to know who my true friends were. How can I not be consumed by all this, I will forever be changed.

I forwarded the latest report from the radiologist to our naturopathic dr We'd had a lot of trouble getting this report, as the doctor hadn't wanted us to have it. Perhaps he knew we were going for a second opinion and would find the biopsy he'd suggested was unwarranted.

In addition, I informed our naturopath that our urologist had concluded from Perry's clear and negative urine analysis in November that because the previous one in October hadn't been clear, the latest one didn't rule out that one as highly suspicious of malignancy. How could that be? Was the doctor being unreasonable? Didn't the second test result indicate we were making progress? These were the questions that needed to be addressed and the reason we needed a second opinion and some good advice about the truth of Perry's current condition.

Perry had no pain, no difficulty urinating, and no blood present in his urine. He felt well and certainly looked well, although he was stressed now, given that our doctor refused to acknowledge that what we were doing was at least keeping the cancer from progressing.

I'd also researched and read that a kink in the ureter can also be congenital, and the natural out-pouching he'd been born with in his bladder could also cause a natural distension in the ureter. It was all getting a bit much for me to cope with, but my instincts were telling me not to trust this doctor any longer. Ureter surgery could go wrong and the ureter could wind up permanently damaged.

The urologist also told us he didn't have the equipment to remove a tumour from the ureter. He only had the equipment to do a biopsy of a suspected tumour. This in turn made me very suspicious of his ability.

If Perry did have a tumour in the ureter, then surely we needed to first find another urologist—someone who had the correct equipment and team of doctors and could remove it and not just take a slice of it.

## 10 January

The appointment with the naturopath didn't go the way I'd wanted. I'd been hoping the radiologist would be there to look at the MRIs for us, but she wasn't. All we were able to do was have another urine cytology and routine blood tests to determine whether we'd successfully managed Perry's previous vitamin deficiency.

Our naturopath did tell us that, if Perry had a tumour in his ureter, then it would definitely have shown up in the most recent urine cytology. She said all of the markers were negative and remarked how great Perry was looking. She was more concerned with how stressed I was now. She recommended some natural serotonin for me and also said she thought we would be better off seeing another urologist rather than just having someone look at the MRIs.

We now had to wait until Perry returned from a trip to Egypt for him to see another urologist. But we would get the results from his blood and urine tests on Sunday or Monday.

I'd been thinking a lot more clearly again now. I knew the immune system was a never-ending second-by-second check of all your cells to see if they still acted like they always did. So why had I been letting the negative feedback from the doctor affect my thoughts in such a profound way?

I was back to my research, as it was my only comfort. Reading the testimonies of thousands of people and doctors who believed natural healing could occur if you treated your body right and gave it the help it needed to heal itself gave me the strength to believe in what we were doing.

Research showed that, in a normal body, hundreds of potential cancer cells appeared every day. These defective mutated cells were usually destroyed by the normal immune system and never caused a problem. Cancer only got started when a failing immune system began to allow abnormal cells to slip by without triggering an attack on them.

Looking at it this way, a tumour was a symptom of a failing immune system. Perry's immune system was now in peak condition, and hopefully, the blood tests we'd done today would prove this. If this proved to be the case, we'd be foolish to go ahead and compromise his immune system by having a biopsy when he had no pain and no problem, simply because of what a doctor thought he might have seen on an MRI.

Most cancers never cause any symptoms, and early screening often leads to unnecessary treatment. The immune system can hold many problems in check, as long as it is not compromised by invasive procedures. Our bodies have a powerful ability to encapsulate altered tissue areas, indefinitely.

It's this exact natural mechanism of protective encapsulation that is disregarded by conventional medicine whenever cancer is suspected. We have to biopsy it, the doctors say, to see whether or not it's cancerous. And immediately! But why?

First of all, by the time any lump is big enough to be detected, it has usually been there for at least a year, maybe several. So what's the rush? Why not see how your body handles it. If it remains unchanged over time, chances are the encapsulation can eventually be resorbed, or at least permanently walled off. These common-sense notions are simply not entertained, not deemed worthy of consideration by the specialists. Doctors will say anything to frighten you until you agree to get the biopsy. We are not allowed to get too comfortable with the notion that, the more time goes by without treatment, the better we feel—or that the body actually has powerful resources of healing all of its own.

Perry's doctor was amazed I'd even thought of this. He smiled when I told him what I knew and then sternly told me it had not been scientifically proven! That the tumour could be encapsulated. Then he went to extreme lengths to convince us that the body didn't have this power of walling off invaders and tumours.

## 11 January

Following any advice from someone who had again stated that the only cure for Perry was to remove his bladder, ureter and prostate, even though the test results clearly showed improvement and regression in the thickening of the muscle of the bladder was, to say the least, difficult. Our urologist wouldn't even acknowledge the improvements. He again told us that no scientific evidence suggested that the reduced thickening of the wall was a good sign.

This doctor laid out what would likely happen if we didn't do as he said. Once again, he gave Perry one to two years to live. No doubt, he wouldn't put that in writing if we asked him to. If this was the case, then Perry had already used up six months of his time, and he'd never felt fitter or healthier.

It was definitely time for us to start looking around for a second opinion and our third urologist. I had to see if I could find alternative solutions to our situation that had a little sunnier outlook. It was a big world out there.

It was this same initiative that had led me to investigate natural cures in the first place. My intuition was working overtime now, and I learned about so many programs that didn't include words like *terminal* and *side effects* and *expiration date* and *cell death*.

Over the last few days, my husband and I have both experienced how much power a thought could have—how much impact negative people and negative input could have. Such a constantly degrading social pattern could lead to abnormal changes at the cellular level as a result of stress. We now also had to remove ourselves from negative things and people, especially if those negative forces be family members.

We'd been lucky. We only really had one family member who disagreed with our protocol. This naysayer had retired from a medical profession. And had a total disregard for any type of alternative healing

If you're going to try a program like the one we'd chosen, don't be naïve enough to expect everyone's approval. Expect ridicule. I'd already encountered plenty of that.

Avoid those people who offer ridicule, no matter who they are. Is this selfish? You bet. It's time to be selfish.

The greatest difficulty in a holistic program for cancer is not the discipline required by the program itself. Neither is it the time it requires, the money involved, or the newness of the lifestyle. The biggest obstacle is the solitude of it all. I felt like I was canoeing upstream, without a paddle.

This was one time in our life when it was okay to upset people— the one time it was fine to be completely selfish. We all have a right to our own life, no matter how politically incorrect that notion becomes.

If you find out you have cancer, then it seems to me you've got one chance. Go for it 100 per cent—diet, detox, take supplements, do major cardio exercise, and eliminate all negative input. Start immediately and it will work. Document everything.

I had to stop wasting energy thinking I had to learn enough to convince these geniuses that they may be wrong and there may be another way. It wasn't in their professional DNA to even consider alternatives, and it was clear they'd spent zero time researching alternative treatments. People who choose the holistic path seriously inform themselves and then make up their own minds.

## 13 January

My husband was on his way to Egypt for business. It had been a terrible few days for us both, and for the first time in six months, Perry had begun to show signs of being under severe stress!

On Friday morning, he told me he had something he needed to tell me. He'd passed a large blood clot in his urine on Thursday and again on Friday, just one big one and one small one. He said he'd had no pain before or during the passing. But he needed to tell me because he knew the urine analysis he'd had on Thursday would come back positive for blood cells. He knew he would be away when I got the results, so he needed to tell me before the doctor called.

We both went through a lot of scenarios. Maybe the clot was what was showing up on the MRI and now it had come out naturally, and on and on. We both hadn't slept all night. He told me he felt better now that he'd told me, as he'd considered keeping this from me. But he hadn't wanted me to panic when I got the results.

Later in the day, I got the results we'd been waiting for by email. As predicted, the blood work showed high counts of red blood cells in his urine again, which could indicate a number of things. I emailed the naturopath and told her about the blood clots. She had no answers for me. She could only suggest that Perry have another MRI to see if a kidney stone was the cause. She suggested that, for now, Perry should take the antibiotics he'd bought before he left and drink plenty of water. Then we should ask for a scan when we saw the new urologist on Perry's return on Saturday.

Perry has been taking mega doses of vitamin D at the naturopath's recommendations. But I'd just read that high levels of vitamin D could cause kidney stones, as well as high pH levels. Perry had been taking bicarbonate of soda to raise his pH, but his level had come back at 9, far too high and much higher than his usual reading of 8. I'd also just read that, not only can low acidic pH levels cause kidney stones, so can pH levels that are extremely high (over 8). Perhaps the blood in his urine was caused by a kidney stone that he'd finally passed. All we could do was cling to the hope that this was the answer and remember that, other than feeling a little stressed, Perry was doing well. He continued to feel no pain, had no visible blood in his urine, and said he felt well.

I was desperate for him to return home so we could go and speak with a new urologist. I hoped the new doctor would be able to give him a scan the same day. And I was anxious for him to have another urine test, now that he'd taken the antibiotics; perhaps he'd just had another infection, and all would be well with another test.

I had an email today from our naturopath. She urged me to inform Perry to stop taking his vitamin D immediately, as his levels were far too high. The appropriate levels for treating cancer were 70 to 100, and his were around 125. In addition, his DHEA levels were high too.

We had to make another appointment with her. I needed to discuss what I'd read about elevated pH levels causing kidney stones.

Perry said he felt fine and had no visible blood in his urine. He would return Thursday evening from Egypt.

## Saturday, 19 January

I was losing my ability to function properly. I felt defeated and worried sick as I wondered what the new urologist would tell us. But I knew we had to have another opinion, as somehow I didn't trust what we'd been told by the head radiologist at the last hospital. I felt we were being persuaded by scare tactics yet again to have yet another biopsy. It was just a hunch, but it was a gut-wrenching hunch. And we just couldn't take the chance that it was right.

The power our own thoughts have over us amazed me. That power here had never been more obvious than it had this past week. I couldn't think straight or smile, and tears were never too far away.

A friend of ours gave us the name of a German urologist who spoke perfect English. He made us feel very welcome and comfortable and took his time to explain everything. I'd been so worried about going over everything again with yet another doctor who I presumed wouldn't want to listen to someone embarking on a road of natural healing. But I could not have been more wrong.

This doctor listened to us for at least thirty minutes and asked various questions. Then he said, "No doctor has the power to say something will not work or that, if you do not go down a certain road, you will die." He told us a story of a young man who had more or less been given a death sentence after being diagnosed with a terrible sinus cancer. This person went the alternative route and was now cancer free and having his first child. The doctor explained that, as a carer, I should also take better care of myself, as what we were undertaking is all-psychological and it affected the entire family unit.

I'd forgotten to look after myself. I knew I needed to relax more and smile more, but how could I?

This kind thoughtful man and Dr looked through all the latest MRI scans and explained everything in detail to us. He showed us that Perry's right kidney wasn't inflamed; it had merely split into almost two congenitally (as he'd developed in his mother's womb). He said the out-pouching of the bladder was also congenital. In addition, he explained that the kink in Perry's ureter could also be a result of the birth defect, explaining that, as Perry had never previously had any problems, these defects weren't discovered until he'd had these MRIs. Finally, he told us that he could see no mass and no cancer in the bladder. Nor could he see enough thickening of the ureter wall to warrant a biopsy. He said there was no reason to put the body through a four-hour procedure with anaesthetic to take a look inside the bladder when he could do this with a local anaesthetic and a cystoscopy in his clinic.

Words couldn't describe how this made us feel; I was smiling from ear to ear and extremely happy for the first time in such a long while.

The doctor went on to recommend nothing more invasive than a cystoscopy every three months to make sure no seeds of cancer were growing. If he found any growing cells, he would prescribe BCG along with some laser treatments to keep the cancer at bay.

He asked about urine cytology and fount through our records that Perry had never had a tumour marker done. He said this test would tell him immediately whether any cancer cells were present.

He did the urine test, and twenty minutes later, he told us the test was negative.

Perry was elated; he told me he was shaking with joy. I kissed him and told him, "We did it!" Today was a fantastic day and we needed to celebrate.

I wrote this on my family face book

> OMG—cannot keep this to myself and cannot wait
> and take time to write private messages, so I am
> doing it publicly. Perry is cancer free at this moment.
> He has no cancer visible on the MRI and scan and
> no cancer cells in his urine and no reason to have
> another biopsy. We found another urologist, and he
> said he only needs a follow-up cystoscopy every three
> months because of his history! Thank God I listened
> to my intuition. His cancer—free state is official, but
> he'll have to be monitored until the five-year mark.
> I am one happy lady.

## 21 January

Yesterday, we cancelled the scheduled biopsy. We were now waiting for the first urologist to question us as to why we'd made this decision.

Perry had to okay this new urologist and his plan to be monitored via a cystoscopy every three months with the insurance company. Then we could schedule his first cystoscopy in the very near future. And hopefully, we could relax for three months, in the knowledge that what we were doing is working and Perry was being monitored by a doctor who was open to our methods of treatment.

## 23 January

The first cystoscopy was now booked for Saturday. We were anxious, but it had to be done. All the nagging it took to get him to book in for this exploratory procedure was draining. Perry was of the mind that he was cancer free, so we should just keep doing what we were doing. But I knew we couldn't take the chance that the cancer might come back We had to have regular check-ups to make sure nothing was developing, so that, if it came back, we'd have the opportunity to stop it in its tracks.

Our new Urologist had advised that Perry have this procedure every three months, and it had been six months since his last biopsy, which gave his doctors an actually view inside the bladder, rather than just on the scans or MRIs. Yes it was nerve-racking, but the urine cytology had been negative and nothing had been visible on MRI. So now was a good time to start the regular checks.

## 25 January

The cystoscopy was scheduled for tomorrow, and Perry was nervous. I could tell because he was snappy. He wanted to just forget about all we'd endured and believe he was cured, as if he'd had a bad case of flu. But sadly, it didn't work like that, and these regular check-ups had to be done.

I'd realized that I'd been consumed with his illness and was probably not fun to be around. But I was certainly finding out who my true friends were, and that was a blessing in itself.

One of the most important things you need in order to make your goals a reality is a strong support system of like-minded, *positive* people! If people who dismiss you or fill your head with negative chatter surround you, these "friends" can hold you back more than you may realize. (I'm not saying you should stop seeing these friends! But I do believe you should limit the amount of time you spend with people who bring you down and spend more time with those who lift you up and will help support you on your journey.

I'd learned not to take it personally when someone is negative towards what we were trying to achieve. Someone else's negativity often has absolutely nothing to do with you! Instead, it's usually their issue. So just let negative comments go in one ear and out the other!

Remember that you are in control of your own life. No matter what others may say, you are ultimately in charge of your thoughts.

So remember, when others start to make you feel down, you have the power to turn it around and pick yourself back up.

## 26 January

I was disappointed today. We couldn't have cystoscopy because a mix-up with Perry's appointment date meant the equipment wasn't sterile. We rebooked for Tuesday.

He had psyched himself up to get the procedure done, and it was disappointing. But we did get some positive news from the doctor. He informed us that the urine cytology had come back from the path lab as negative for any presence of malignancy, bacteria, or blood. He reconfirmed that whatever we were doing was working and that all the cystoscopy was for was to check the cells in Perry's bladder; the exam would reveal either dead cancer cells or dormant inactive cells, or, in the best-case scenario, he'd find only normal, healthy cells. In the end, though we were a little disappointed we could not find out today, we also felt very happy.

How scary it was to think that the route to this recovery was a gentle restoring of the body using Perry's immune system, rather than the toxic destruction that seemed to be inevitable with the methods generally used in our health care system.

## 29 January

Today we had the cystoscopy. The doctor let me look inside Perry's bladder to see for myself that he'd found a small tumour. He wanted me to describe it to him in my own words so he could explain what it meant in terms of cancer.

Bladder cancer that's at an early stage of growth may not produce any noticeable signs. That was why neither the MRI nor the urine cytology had alerted us to this tumour. We'd caught it this time before it showed these signs.

He said the tumour had to be removed and, knowing the path we'd chosen, gave us a few options for doing this. The first option, as far as a surgeon was concerned, would be to completely remove the bladder. (He knew this was not an option for us.) The second option would be to scrape the tumour and do a biopsy, but this could release cancer cells, as it would leave the wound open to heal. The third option was to avoid a biopsy altogether, as the cancer was not releasing cells—this was why the urine cytology had shown up negative—and simply laser the entire thing off and seal the wound so that nothing was open. Then we could either do radiation (again not an option for us) or BCG medicine through a catheter into the bladder every week for four to six weeks. After that, we'd do another cystoscopy to check how it had worked. Our fourth and final option was to do nothing; the tumour would either remain dormant (not releasing cells) or it could grow.

We had a big decision to make again. We trusted this doctor and felt he was honest. He showed me clearly that there was something in Perry's bladder.

We both decided that the laser option was the best one for now. As this tumour has been growing there for the last six months without releasing cells into the bladder, we didn't need to rush into things. The body has a powerful ability to encapsulate altered tissue areas, indefinitely. This cancer wasn't showing up in any tests, so something in his immune system was working.

We were due to go to England this month for ten days for our granddaughter's christening, so we decided to wait until we returned. We would then decide whether Perry wanted any further treatment (BCG) after the laser treatment or whether to simply continue with what we were doing. We feel that what we were doing was keeping the cancer at bay, even if it hadn't completely disappeared. Perry said that he was listening to his own body. He felt very well and didn't want to compromise this with harsh treatments of any kind. But to have the tumour lasered couldn't do much harm, and then it would be gone.

I was researching all over again. I felt okay all day, unlike when we'd been with the last doctor. I had never trusted him. And now I'd seen the tumour for myself. Our new doctor had let me be involved in the cystoscopy, and I'd seen it clearly with my own eyes. I even knew what kind of cancer it was, as I'd done so much research.

The urologist hadn't said why it had grown, but I could only imagine it was a result of the biopsy six months early. That procedure had left the wound open to heal and release cells. But luckily, what we were doing had halted it from spreading. It hadn't been enough to stop that particular tumour from growing back though.

I decided we had to look on the positive side and be happy that the cancer hadn't spread to another site or organ and had just grown back. At this stage, we didn't know how large it was, but it wasn't very big. We could only hope and pray that it would shrink and disappear or just not become active. But I believed we'd both feel better once it was removed and as we kept an eye on the site, going in for a check-up every three months.

That proved easier said than done, as I found out when we went to bed and the pains in my chest started again. I was having another anxiety attack, so I had to get up as I had done so many nights. Perry was sleeping, which was a good thing, and I was again alone with my thoughts and my research.

## 1 February

We were literally being ripped apart emotionally. I was consumed with feelings of guilt. Maybe it was my fault that the cancer had come back. Maybe I should have done more.

We were constantly getting pulled back and forth; we'd experience manic happiness at being told no cancer could be found, and then came the darkness of fear that had once again reared its ugly head.

We had so much happiness and peace and strength of conviction; we could laugh and enjoy our beautiful life together most of the time.

But then there were so many times lately when we were both so overwhelmed with stress and fear that we were snappy with each other. We were both consumed by everything we were dealing with, and *it* though we didn't talk about it—what if he doesn't make it?—Was a constant presence we were both aware. It was on the faces of family and friends who were trying to be supportive and in their words and voices on telephone calls.

Fear was everywhere. But all this was making us even more determined to win this battle. It was the force that had driven us in the direction of alternative healing. We were only just learning that, as hard as the diagnosis was for us to bear in the beginning, it wasn't the worst we'd felt in the last six months.

As we tried to get on with our lives, dazed but determined, I had such a powerful intuition that the path we had chosen was the only way. One path led us to conventional cancer treatments—chemotherapy, radiation, and surgery. The doctors told us it would surely be a cure, but now our new urologist had told us that no doctor could guarantee a cure.

Doctors are not gods and do not have all the answers. Think about it. That's why physicians have medical "practices." No physician (medical, allopathic, or naturopathic) can guarantee a "cure," and "remission" is not the same thing as a "cure". Chemotherapy uses powerful drugs to "kill" the cancer cells, but they also destroy the body's God-given immune system. With or without allopathic medical treatment or complementary alternative natural treatment, there simply are no guarantees regarding the successful cure of the disease. A person's own mental outlook on the success of treatment (or not) can greatly affect the treatment's outcome.

Whilst our method of treatment was keeping Perry looking and feeling healthy and happy most of the time and certainly at the moment it was a painless option for him. The cancer had still returned, our urologist had tried to put us at ease. He'd told us that, given that Perry had gone for six months without receiving chemotherapy or radiation, he'd have expected the cancer to be more aggressive than before. In my opinion, if he'd undergone chemo and radiation, the cancer would surely have metastasized, as his immune system, depleted by the aggressive conventional treatment, would have been unable to fight the spread of the cancer.

This eased our worries a little. Perry's immune system was the strongest it had ever been, owing to the natural treatments he was taking and the diet and lifestyle changes he had adopted. This new finding didn't daunt us. We were just ready for another chance to prove that the path we'd chosen was the right path for him.

## 2 February

Perry left yesterday for another trip to Egypt. He called me from the airport and said he was sorry he'd been snappy. He said he was sorry a lot lately! Physically he was well, but mentally, he must be stressed.

He had been elated to choose this path. The idea of radiation and chemotherapy and, worst of all, having his bladder and prostate removed haunted him. So once we'd decided to take the path we were on, I'd seen instant elation. He'd felt as if life had something to offer him. This was even before we knew what we were going to do; just the thought of not having to go the expected and traditional route was enough to lift his spirits.

That, coupled with my intuition that this was the right choice, had brought us so close and united as a couple. Yet recent events had altered that slightly. Perry had to face yet another surgery (which he didn't want to do), and he also had a lot of work at the moment. So he couldn't deal with me asking questions about whether he'd taken this vitamin or ran out of anything. I had to try to back off a little. I didn't have a job, so my full-time focus was concentrated on getting him well—assessing how he was feeling, feeding him properly, and generally being there for him.

I figured this break would do us both good. I would concentrate on my art, and he will get on with his work without interruption from me.

# 5 February

Today I received a beautiful e-mail from my son's friend's mum and former teacher, who had asked to read my journal. It bought a tear to my eye, and I wanted to share it.

> The note,
>
> I remember meeting you many years ago at a parent-teacher conference for Kyle when he was at school and I was privileged to teach him.
>
> I never thought our boys would become such great friends and that you and I would connect again in such a significant way. This is how God works. Nothing is ever a coincidence—I was meant to read your journal today! And wow . . . You are a truly amazing woman. I feel so inspired. Your resolve is remarkable!
>
> I would often ask Kyle about his parents, and the reply was always a "yeah, they're all right." When Nic was in South Africa, he sent me a pic of Kyle in a hospital with his dad. He informed me of his illness, and I sensed the worry in Nic's tone. I met Kyle one day and asked him about his dad. I was visibly shaken by the news. I wanted Kyle to know that we, as a family, were there for him and his family and that I would keep his dad in my prayers. And we

said goodbye. I saw Kyle again when Nic returned in January, and I asked him again about Perry, and with a smile on his face, he shared the great news.

My goodness, what a journey this is for you! Your tenacity and perseverance astounds me. Your courage and strength fragments wars!

I lost a niece in 2010 at the tender age of twenty-eight to lymphatic cancer. Her mom struggles so intensely today to cope with Bronwyns's death, and she continually questions the medication prescribed to Bron. She did admit to me over Christmas, though, that the doctors informed her that it was, indeed, the chemo that destroyed Bronwyn's heart because, in the end, she died because her heart stopped. Needless to say, this was devastating to us as a family. So hats off to you for doing all the research and your unending quest for finding alternative cures.

I will continue to hold you, your sons, daughter-in-law, and grandchildren in my prayers. Yet another powerful means of fostering hope!

All the best and do remember, I am here should you need anything at all okay?

## 10 February

As I got back to my research, I was renewed with positive thoughts surrounding our decision to say no to traditional cancer treatments. What had perked me up was the rates of cancer survival as they are presented to the public are based on five-year increments. That is, if you live for five years after treatment, then the treatment is considered a success. Overall, the survival rates do not specify whether cancer survivors are still undergoing treatment at five years, whether they still have cancer, or whether they've achieved remission. Quality of life is also not factored into the picture. So if you're lying in bed comatose on a morphine drip five years after diagnosis, then the treatment given is still considered a success.

Traditional cancer treatment destroys people; it is so enormously painful and exhausting that it is almost too much for the everyday person to endure. The image that comes to mind when I think of people undergoing chemo and/or radiation is a body nuked at the core and the fires spreading outward. The chemo and/or radiation moves through the system like toxic poison, killing everything it touches, healthy and unhealthy, and utterly destroying the immune system. The side effects are well documented and horrific. Patients' testimonies out there speak of their inability to walk, an overwhelming physical weakness, exhaustion, the inability to take care of themselves or their children, intense nausea, teeth falling out, hair falling out, chemo induced leukaemia, feeling like drain cleaner is running through their veins, achy bones, achy feet, a sense of being cold all the time, and an awful taste in the mouth.

Cancer patients really do need to inform themselves about alternative treatments. This information—information that's been around for a long, long time, but underground—is getting out there. It's not underground any more. I hope that I can be of some small help to someone also feeling they have nowhere to turn except the Internet for this information.

When you are diagnosed with cancer of any kind, you should ask hard questions. In whom do we trust? We alone are responsible for the body God gave us. It is up to us to seek wise council and always check out the authority and basis for what doctors advise us as the recommended treatment; we need to conduct exhaustive research on our own because doctors don't tell us everything we need to know. Often, the conventional doctor simply doesn't have the extensive training and scientific backgrounds that integrative Doctors who give us the alternative to conventional treatments have. We decided to say no to our conventional doctors, and it is okay for you to say no too.

We do not know of anyone who said yes to conventional treatment and, one month later, felt like he or she was twenty-one again. Perry did physically, and we would continue on this journey and document his progress so that, hopefully one day, we could help others to have the courage to say no too.

# CHAPTER 6

## LASER SURGERY

### 24 February

The laser surgery went well today, but unexpectedly, the doctor found at least twenty small tumours in the out-pouching of his bladder on the right-hand side. He thought by the visual he had had of them that they were all going to be superficial. In addition he couldn't say whether they'd always been there or whether they were new growths and not spotted on the MRI or by the other two surgeons, who had both looked inside his bladder whilst he was under anaesthetic.

This doctor today looked everywhere while he had Perry under anaesthetic, and he recorded it all on a disc for us to actually see for ourselves. He managed to completely remove all the tumours with the laser, and it was pretty gruesome to watch. But we were very glad we could see for ourselves what was actually going on inside Perry. We would continue to be guided through each investigation from here on in with a DVD of all that had been done.

It was a waiting game yet again for a biopsy of the samples. We were both a little dazed, but something was keeping my hopes up, so I felt is my intuition kicking in again and letting me know he was going to be all right.

## 25 February

We made it back home, and Perry was in a little discomfort but nothing major. He was doing well. He'd had the catheter removed, and we'd actually visited the doctor's surgery just a day after his surgery. This in itself showed how strong and well he was, considering he'd had so many tumours removed.

The doctor showed us the video first in his office so he could explain everything to us. We were both shocked to see at least twenty, maybe more, tumours removed. They looked different from the one in the bladder, so we were hoping they were superficial. It was great to finally see for us what the doctor did and what to look for next time.

We were both left a little numb as to what to think and confused. Why hadn't the other doctors seen these tumours? Why hadn't they shown up on the MRI or in the urine and blood tests?

At least they'd now been discovered and, hopefully, all removed so we could start all over again, trying to build his immune system back up.

The doctor advised Perry to return in eight weeks' time for another laser procedure, during which he'd check for new growths and clean up the area. That way, he could be sure the growths had been completely eradicated. After that, we would need to come back every three months for a visual examination. But we were hoping for some good news after the biopsy. We'd get the results on 3 March.

# CHAPTER 7

## AN ILLEGAL TREATMENT

### Saturday, 2 March

Last year in October or November, I had come across a woman called Corrie Yelland on Facebook when I was researching cannabis oil and the cure for cancer. I read her story on how she'd cured her anal canal cancer (the same form of cancer that killed Farah Fawcett) using the Rick Simpson oil from the video *Run from the cure*

Since finding Corrie on Facebook, I'd had some great chats with her, and she suggested that Perry and I Skype with her, which we did. We spoke at length about her experience and also about where we could get the oil. We told her our predicament, explaining that we didn't dare risk bringing it here to the Middle Eastern country where we were living.

Corrie was very helpful and full of information about the best places to get the oil She suggested we go back to the UK for around three months so Perry could take the oil there and said she could have it mailed to us from the United States. She was a wonderful person to talk to!

When Corrie first told her doctors she was going to use the oil instead of accepting conventional chemo and radiation treatments, they told her she had a "death wish." The following is one of her posts on Facebook about her own story:

> I saw my primary GP this morning. He was a doctor who was dead set against cannabis use on any level. A few months ago, he covered his ears, saying "La, la, la, la, la" when I tried to tell him I was using cannabis oil to fight my cancer. Today, as the doctor who has seen his terminal patient emerge cancer free after using cannabis oil, he has done a 180 [degree] turn and has been researching the heck out of cannabinoids and disease conditions. We talked for 30 minutes or so, discussing the endocannabanoid system, how pharmaceuticals are killing people every day, the ludicrous thoughts of making drugs like Sativex when one can take it in a plant form without chemical involvement. He spoke of my surgeon, at a medical convention he had recently been to, and me—how they were telling their colleagues about me, about cannabanoids! He said they "were spurned by many" but that there were also doctors who paused, listened, and that one could see their wheels turning. Never in a million years did I think my doctor would *ever* come around to this! Yes, one person *can* make a difference! Get the word out, peeps. *Cannabis kills cancer.*

After talking with Corrie and a few more days of research, Perry and I decided that our next step had to involve the oil. We looked into making arrangements to spend some time in England, possibly for three months, once we had the oil ready and the instructions for using it.

## 3 March

Today we got the results from the biopsy, which were good and bad. The good news was that all the tumours that had been removed were superficial tumours, which meant they hadn't invaded the muscle and there was no lymph node involvement or vesicle metastasis. The cancer was still contained within the bladder, but at this moment in time it has not progressed further.

This was fantastic news for us, but we had to be mindful that, because multiple tumours had been removed, this was considered to be aggressive superficial cancer and highly likely to recur. Although that didn't have to be the case, it did, however, mean that we had to be vigilant about keeping follow-up procedures with the surgeon and getting regular cystoscopies to check his bladder for recurrences.

## 4 March

First, I would like to stress that both my husband and I were completely against the use of drugs. Neither of us had ever taken any form of drugs, for recreation or any other reason, other than those prescribed to us by doctors for medical reasons. Now, we'd both had a complete change of heart and were doing what we could to get the illegal cannabis oil medicine from Amsterdam.

All we knew was that we had to do whatever we could to ensure that Perry's cancer was eradicated once and for all and to do it while he was strong and well if that was possible.

The treatment involves cannabis oil that's derived from cannabis plant and is, therefore, illegal in the UK and most of the world.

We had to get a ninety-day course of treatment from a medical marijuana pharmacy in Amsterdam. I was extremely worried about collecting it, and I'd been in touch with a few people who'd told me it is possible to get it posted to England. We were in the process of finding out whether that was the case.

First, a woman in Canada informed me she had a contact in the United States who would ship the cannabis oil to me in the United Kingdom. Then this contact told me a partner in Amsterdam would sort out the order for me. I got in touch with her, and she informed me it would be best that we came to collect it. The cost would be just over 2,000 pounds for sixty grams (the amount Perry would need for a period of three months). I emailed this woman back to tell her I was too nervous to collect it and wanted to know if it was possible to get it posted. I asked her to please advise me, letting her know that, if I had to collect it, I would. I was waiting anxiously for her reply.

## 7 March

I received a reply from Amsterdam, stating again that I should go there and post our order of the oil to an address in the United Kingdom. She told me I could pack it in a way that would be suitable for shipping and, on its arrival, repack it into syringes for dispensing.

I was still uncomfortable with this set-up and continued to scour the Internet for a UK contact. I looked through many sites, but I stumbled upon one that stuck out from the rest. Bud Buddies, a UK-based British organization, had been supplying cannabis for medicinal use from 2002 to 2007. Now they were researching the preparation and application of cannabis oil.

The company overview stated, "Bud Buddies are currently researching cannabinoid concentrated oil. Our oils are produced in Spain and UK. However, we do not sell or supply commercially." They are a select group of likeminded individuals who are devoted to producing and evaluating the medicinal benefits of cannabis oil.

When I first had a look at the site, I came across a remark suggesting that patients who were waiting should grow their own cannabis, as the company could only help a handful of people a year. In addition, they take new patients on to assist their research. The note also explained that, later this year, Bud Buddies would be helping with oil preparations and documenting their progress. The website noted that a particular person would be setting up an experimental medical grow room as well as making the oils the company sold, adding that it was going to be an exciting year. I wrote to Bud Buddies explaining our situation and asked for some help. Within ten minutes, I got a reply:

> Hi, sorry to hear your news. We recommend that cancer sufferers who wish to use the therapy should grow their own cannabis. However, in your country, I wouldn't even suggest you have it in your possession. I'm sure you will get someone to provide you with the oil; the problem is though that there are people out there selling fake and sub-standard oil. The oil makers in the US and Amsterdam don't have their oils tested. We are lucky because all ours are and they're also made correctly. What's your husband's prognosis?

We wrote back and forth for a while, until eventually, I decided to go to Spain and collect some oil from a contact my contact at Budd Buddies gave me there. All the while, I was feeling nervous. But I knew I needed to do this for my husband.

I started making plans to go to Spain. One of my sisters assured me she would go with me. I told her I would love to have some company while I was there to help me get to the right place and at least feel a little support whilst doing this illegal purchase, but I insisted that I would come back with the medicine alone. This was a serious business, and it broke my heart to know that this oil—a God-given plant medicine—could be the answer for so many people who were suffering and that their loved ones would have to break the law to get their hands on it.

## 8 March

Our visit to the doctor today was very interesting. He told us about a new treatment he had to offer Perry—for the first time ever in this part of the world.

A special type of laser light called photodynamic therapy was focused on the inner lining of the bladder through a cystoscope. The light allows the viewer to see the cancer before the naked eye could. The surgeon would then zap the area with a laser and kill the cells before they ever developed.

The advantage of PDT was that it could kill cancer cells with no harm to normal cells.

## 15 March

So much had happened over the last two weeks. I'd spent many days talking with lots more people. I made the mistake I'd shared my thoughts and intentions with close family and friends, and I'd gotten very mixed views. I'd received messages and emails from my mother and sister, who were obviously extremely worried about me going to fetch the oil and bring it through customs myself. In addition, one of my sisters stressed that no one would even want me to post it to their address!

Then I got many messages like this one . . .

Alyssia

You have balls the size of the moon!!! You took them on, and you were right. I'm going to always trust my instincts from now on and always look for alternatives when something doesn't feel right. I want to possess moon balls in exchange for my tiny mustard seed ones. I am such a *yes* person, even when I know things just aren't quite right!!!!! You've changed my mindset. Oh Lord, wow—this is truly amazing. I've managed to share the links on my page. Hope it stays on there because I know Big Brother likes to keep an eye on us, and God forbid if we ever uncover the truth. Keep doing what you are doing and God bless you, my angel. xxxx and more kisses xxxx

Messages like this last one from a friend made me cry and also made me realize how strong I really was and what I was capable of. I always said that I loved the way I was. But then confidence would get clouded when I'd get overwhelmed by all that we were doing. Messages like this really helped me see myself in a different light.

After many more nights of lost sleep, I had again plucked up the courage to go and pick up the oil. I wondered how I would dare go and bring in an illegal substance. Each person I talked to told me I could go and just post it to myself in the United Kingdom or bring it through myself.

My husband was talking to his boss to ask if he could work from England so he could continue his treatment with alternative medicine, as our newest phase of therapy wasn't allowed in this country.

Even whilst I was making these plans and had, eventually, sourced the oil, something was telling me to carry on looking. And so I continued to scour the Internet for a way to get the cannabis oil into the United Kingdom without having to go and bring it in myself. I'd had many interesting conversations, some not so helpful, with people all over the world. I'd spent countless hours on the Internet, scouring sites of cannabis activists for clues as to where to find this healing oil, as well as medical sites to inform myself that what I'd learned was true.

I eventually found a woman who was a natural healing practitioner in California, where cannabis was legal if used for medical purposes. She had various websites that I researched for days before contacting her. I asked for her help, and we Skyped a few times so she could explain what she did and how she had helped heal many sick people with the oil. Her husband (an herbalist) made the oil himself and it was thoroughly tested for potency and made in a clinical way.

Throughout all of our conversations, this practitioner stressed to me that diet was the best way forward to treating many illnesses. I explained all we'd been doing and told her I had kept a journal. She was impressed and wanted to read it. She said it was fantastic and that she wished more people would do this, as documenting everything was helpful for future reference and because it would allow people to look back and see what they'd achieved with different treatments.

She was also very interested in all the information about Essiac. After reading my journal, she did some research herself about these herbs. Now, she wanted to start making this herbal remedy for her patients. She expressed her enthusiasm about having this information from me and told me that this, along with Perry's diet and lifestyle changes, was probably already curing him.

She also sent me this lovely message:

> You absolutely have the makings of a brilliant book!!
> I appreciate you sharing it. Too bad we are twelve
> hours apart. Sleep well now. It's all-good, and this will
> arrive safely, and the last piece of this nasty invasion
> into your husband's life will be gone!

We had ordered the oil and gotten detailed instructions on how Perry was to take it. The California practitioner told me it would come from her legitimate essential oil business and would be packaged as a health product. We would also get a receipt for oil as a health and beauty product.

All this worry and research had finally paid off, and we should receive the oil in about two weeks now. We were now making plans to stay in the United Kingdom for up to three months, so that Perry could take this medicine.

## 16 March

The information was out there. We just needed to know where to look and have the passion to do it. I was once again pondering where we would be without the Internet. I wouldn't have been able to do all the research I'd done or contact all the amazing people who'd inspired me. So I gave thanks today for the computer, Facebook, and my enquiring mind. I had learned to never stop believing in what I was doing and that to be inspired was a good thing but to inspire someone else was a great achievement.

## 18 March

Perry received word today that he could work from England for up to three months. This was great news for us. All we had to do now was decide when to go, and that would depend on two things—first, that the medicine arrived safely in two weeks' time and, second, what the doctor found on 7 April, when Perry was to get his next cystoscopy and laser light treatment. If the test detected no signs of new growths, then we would be able to relax and head for England; Perry would take the cannabis oil in June, July, and August. If, however, the doctor found new growths, we would go home as soon as we could to start on the medicine.

## 28 March

Today was a momentous day; our package arrived safely in England. Today was the beginning of our journey with the oil. We could now relax and decide when to take three months away from the Middle East. I was filled with happiness.

I had started worrying about whether the package would arrive. I'd had nightmares that the police would go to the delivery address. But no problems had arisen. The oil had arrived in two jars, just as the practitioner in California had said it would with essential oils packaging.

My sister sent me a photo of it, and my mum couldn't believe we'd paid so much money for two jars of oil But they didn't know how important these two little jars were, how much sleep had been lost over them, or how hard this was for me to finally purchase and have posted to England.

## 6 April

We had a visit to the doctor's office this morning, owing to the fact that we, once again, ran into troubles with the insurance company. This time, Perry's insurer wouldn't cover the laser fibre needed for this operation at the hospital the doctor chose. We would now have to wait until he found a new hospital—a facility where the entire procedure and fibre would be covered as a package.

We talked with the doctor about the medicine we planned on Perry taking, and he agreed that, if we just did a cystoscopy before we went, then at least he could see if anything of worry was happening. He could then take time to find the right hospital, and we could do the procedure on our return. (We hoped nothing would be found after Perry had used the cannabis oil.)

I felt that this was the best plan anyway. So we were now looking at returning to England sooner than planned—possibly at the end of this month or next.

# 10 April

I'd become a little overwhelmed with all the information that I'd come across about cannabis oil. It was so much to take in and comprehend. Then I had the burden of translating what I knew to family and friends, which was causing arguments and disagreements. I know what I'd learned was the truth; I felt it with every fibre of my being. But I was knocked sideways when a family member aired negative views around me, especially when this person had done only a little bit of research on the sites that were against this medicine.

I truly believed this was a wonder plant, and I didn't understand how anyone who knew what I now knew could not fight for to legalize the plant so that people could get hold of it and cure themselves. Yes, I understood the politics behind it all. But I was so passionate to get the word out it seemed to have overtaken my every thought. My Facebook page was full of reports people were sending me about the benefits of the oil, testimonials of people who'd cured themselves with it, and articles about this healing plant. Then friends would see the reports and counter-attack with reports on the negative aspects. But these friends hadn't done the research I had, and I couldn't explain what I now knew to be the truth in just a few words. I hadn't set out to be an activist for cannabis oil, but I was fast becoming one. This wasn't my intention. All I ever wanted was to keep my husband well.

Anyone interested in finding most of the information necessary to start your own research into the marijuana plant and its healing powers should read *Marijuana Gateway to Health: How Cannabis Protects Us from Cancer and Alzheimer's Disease* by Clint Werner. In one word,

I would describe this book as brilliant. A quote from Promoter's of the book

"To write a book like this, an author must be a courageous, independent, and discerning investigator with impeccable journalistic integrity. Unfortunately, these qualities are sorely lacking in today's world of investigative reporting. And, unfortunately, the lack of such qualities leads to terrible misinformation, not only about cannabis but about many other "controversial" issues. This book is meticulously researched and intelligently organized, and its content is masterfully distilled, and that allows the reader to easily understand the scientific foundations for the ultimate research conclusions. If everyone read this book, our entire medical establishment would be turned upside down. Or maybe I should say, right side up."

★　★　★

Being supported in what I was doing felt amazing, but lately, I'd felt too much negativity around me. It was such a strong vibration that I'd let it get me down on a few occasions.

I was always able to work better and think better when I was around positive people. Or when I was alone, I would get quiet and create. Painting helped me casting off negative energy.

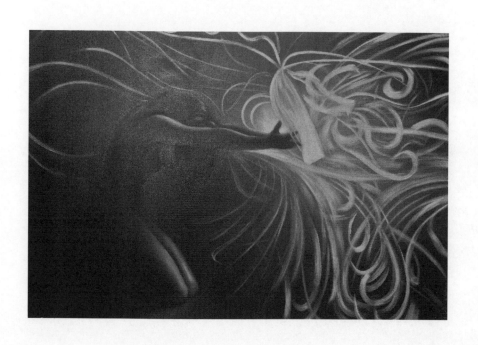

# 14 April

Today I received this beautiful message from a friend after sending her a picture of my latest painting, "Spiritual Awakening." The painting is of a woman reaching up, with light shining from her head. She absolutely put into words what I'd painted, and she bought me to tears with them:

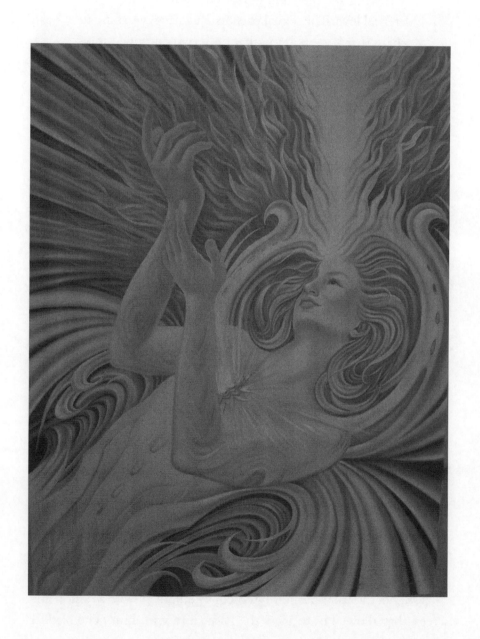

The delicate, fragile image of the female being. Growing and blossoming from the bud that is life and eternal love. The sexual passion. Pulsating, yearning to share that love in a way that only two entwined souls can. Swirls of comfort and peace being disturbed and slightly turbulent. She is a woman, reaching up to God with her spiritual awareness, hands and heart open, cutting off all of the outside world and listening to her spirit inside her. Her sixth sense, her personal message to trust in Him and believe in the beautiful, natural things he has put around us. She is being filled with knowledge, strength and enlightenment. For the love of her man, a love that can never be described in words, the most important thing in her life, he is her life, her being, her soul. Blessed by His Angels to tell her story and share her belief in her sixth self being open and not locked up, like many others who have been covered by the modern system that is the world today. She has given up her fear to Him and smiles slightly as the invisible hand reaches down to her. She is strong. She is beautiful. She is open and free. She has faith.

She is you.

## Saturday, 28 April

Today was Perry's cystoscopy. We couldn't have the laser procedure done, as the insurance wouldn't cover it again. We decided it would be best to get the bladder checked before going to England to take the medical marijuana.

Our doctor had some new cystoscopy equipment with a camera and screen that allowed us to view the procedure with him. The bladder looked healthy and clear, and so did the left-hand side where the natural out-pouching was. But on the right-hand part of the out-pouching where the last twenty or so tumours had been removed by laser, we saw three small growths. The doctor tells us that these were new and that he hadn't miss them during the previous operation. But he told us not to be too concerned. These new growths looked to him to be superficial.

This wasn't good news, but I had to say it certainly wasn't bad. We now had video evidence of what we had to deal with whilst Perry was taking the medicine. And on our return, we would do the same operation to look inside his bladder and see for ourselves at the same time the doctor saw whether the medicine could remove these tumours or stop them from growing.

## Monday, 29 April

So much had been happening to me just lately. I'd become so involved with many people and much more research. I was learning a great deal, and people were coming to me for help. Friends of friends and other people were contacting me daily to ask for advice on diet and medicine. I wanted to help, and I'd been in touch with many; I could link those in need up with the right people.

I'd been following posts from Ian Jacklin, a moviemaker who'd made a documentary called "icurecancer.com". He'd almost completed his second documentary, which would hopefully make it to the major screens. Everything I'd found out about alternative medicine and cures for cancer was covered in Ian's movie, and he'd made it his life's work to get the word out to people.

I was astounded to learn that he'd spent the last fifteen years gathering all this information and he couldn't get a backer for his movie to bring it to the big screen. He was running out of funding and had set up a website with the same name as his film. I'd scoured this site so many times and watched all of his video clips. I felt fortunate as I discovered that we had had already used almost every one of the alternative therapies he recommended, with the exception of the cannabis oil.

Ian had only just come across Cannabis oil as a medicine at a similar time to our own discovery. I was now in contact with him through his Facebook site, and we'd chatted a few times. I felt a compelling urge to help him. He was doing what I would love to do—telling the world that you can say no to traditional treatments. Perry was living proof that alternative therapies worked. I'd spent many nights wondering how I could help Ian.

I realized that a financial donation would be a great way to contribute. However, all we were doing for my husband was costing quite a lot. I asked Perry if we could donate some money, but it was I doing all the research, and he just didn't understand my urgent desire to help others throughout the world listen to their own intuitions.

I decided to sell my beautiful angel painting and donate the proceeds to Ian's cause. I advertised the painting on Facebook and explained what I wanted the money for, and a friend offered to buy it from me for 900 pounds. I donated the money through Ian's website, and being able to help him get this film made felt great. Words couldn't express what being able to do this meant to me.

I received this message from Ian today:

> Oh wow, okay that's amazing 'cause I just ran out of money paying rent today, lol. I was hoping the universe would bring something this way as I would hate to become homeless now that I have the ball rolling so well. This is so kind of you! Someone up there really likes me. Cheers! God bless you!

He told me he would like to use the painting in his movie somewhere and suggested I make the angel painting into a Christmas card, as it was so beautiful. (I thought I would do just that, as I really loved this painting and would miss it so much.)

The painting sort of evolved through all my emotions as I wondered what to do next. When I came across a picture of a stone statue angel with the very same expression I felt, I just had to put it on canvas.

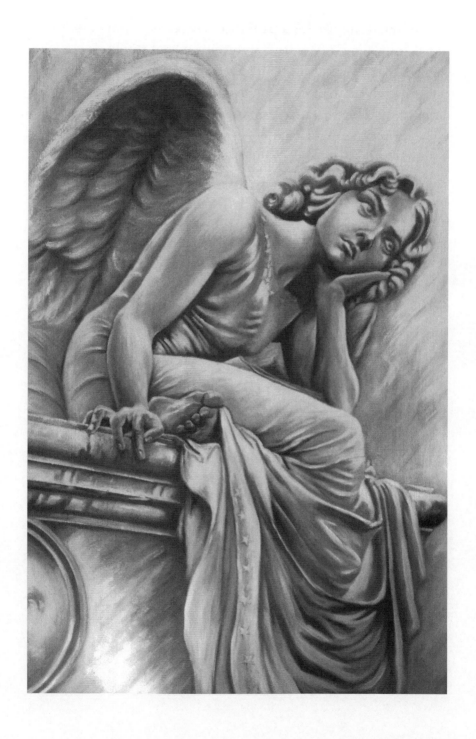

I'd found my feet on a path that was taking me in a direction of self-realization. I wondered if this was what I was meant to do. I seemed to have found what I was put on the earth for—to help others get the word out, to be part of something bigger than what I'd started out to do. I'd never intended to get so involved with other people. I'd never intended for anyone to come to me for advice. I just wanted to find a better way to heal my husband.

I wondered now if this was enlightenment. And in this process and journey, I hoped that perhaps I could inspire others because the fruits and rewards of all of these new experiences were far greater than I could express in words or paint.

# CHAPTER 8
## DARK MONTHS

### 4 May

We'd settled in the apartment in England, and we had the medicine. But my husband wanted to wait until tomorrow to begin his treatment. We had so many people to see today.

I'd decided to keep the journal going every day, in the hope that someone would read the account of our experience and know what to expect. I'd found lots of information about this medicine curing cancer, but nowhere could I find anyone who had documented his or her use of it and its effects. Providing this kind of information would be the purpose of my next three months of entries.

### 5 May

Today, Perry took his first dose of medicine, the size of a grain of rice. He felt no effect after forty minutes so took one other small amount. He still didn't feel any effect. He just went to sleep.

### 6 May

Perry woke this morning feeling like he had a hangover from hell. He was sluggish and couldn't wake himself up. He was not himself.

It was as if he'd had a reaction to anaesthetic. He felt so bad he took himself back to bed and slept for three more hours. It wasn't until around four in the afternoon that he started feeling a little better.

He decided to wait until 7.00 p.m. for his second dose of the day. It was smaller than the doses he'd taken the day before, as we needed to moderate the dosage until he felt he could tolerate more.

I thought his reaction to yesterday's dose was because he had drunk that day as well. You aren't supposed to drink alcohol with this medicine. I wrote to the person from whom I'd gotten the oil, and she recommended a supplement he could take that would help him tolerate the medicine.

We decided to see if he could tolerate one small dose before bedtime and then see how he was on waking tomorrow.

## 7 May

Perry seemed to be tolerating the medicine better today. He woke and took a big dose, followed by another at noon. He did have to have an afternoon nap, but after an hour, he was okay again. The rest would do him good, and hopefully this was all part of the healing process.

Today, I put a one-gram dose into a syringe to see how long it took for Perry to take this amount and to actually see what a gram looked like.

He took one more dose before bedtime and slept for eleven hours, having to go to bed at 9.00 and waking up at 8.00 a.m.

## 8 May

Today, we tried to take the medicine out of the syringe, but it came out too quickly, so Perry took more than he should have. All morning, he looked wiped out, tired, and not completely with it!

He was able to drive, but he was hungrier than normal and had a sort of disinterested look about him all day.

He took a small dose at 3.00 p.m. and went to bed for a couple of hours.

I was worried about him, as he'd never been like this. He was always so bright and full of energy. I understood that this medicine would have this effect on him, but it was so unlike him to have to have a nap in the day.

He was really struggling with the oil. He was still trying to take a little more each day, but it wiped him out. I knew this meant it was the real deal, but it was so unlike him to need a sleep in the day.

## 9th May

This morning, after putting a gram into the syringe, I tried putting a little from the syringe on his finger, but it splodged out more quickly than I'd expected. About three times his normal dosage came out, and it dripped so quickly that he sucked it up, thinking about the cost not wanting to waste the oil. Within an hour, he was acting very strangely! Unresponsive and his conversations were a little distant.

Four hours later, we had an appointment at the gym we had planned to join, and I was sure the assistant thought he was autistic or something. He was so laid-back he tried to put his foot up on my chair to relax, so I quickly pushed it off. I took him home, and he slept for three hours!

Perry really wasn't taking all this too well. The oil had begun to completely wipe him out. I was so used to him being full of energy. If anyone saw him now for the first time, they would think he was ill! He was lethargic and not communicating much at all. He didn't talk unless spoken to, and he just wanted to sit and do nothing.

I wrote to the supplier again, and she advised not to try to get too much inside him too quickly. She told me the medicine was stronger than any other medicine they'd made and she didn't think he'd need the full gram a day.

## 11 May

Today, Perry seemed a little brighter and more himself—until he went out alone to visit his brother after having a small dose. His brother had to drive his car back for him. He said he'd never seen Perry like this before and it worried him, so he wouldn't let him drive. He said he was fine when he arrived, but then he just sat there and said nothing! (Well, he had said he wanted to see his brother, so I suppose he'd done just that.)

Upon returning home, Perry took a small dose and went to bed for three hours again, getting up to eat a huge meal. He seemed okay now if he slept, so we would wait until tonight before giving him a larger dose. He was more himself right now, so I didn't want to give him another dose till bedtime, I needed to feel that we could still talk for at least a few hours a day.

He slept again for eleven hours.

## 12 May

Perry wasn't feeling very well this morning. He had to go back to bed three hours after waking, as he was too tired. The dose he'd taken last night was almost half a gram, and it was only day seven.

He hadn't been very talkative all day, but he seemed relaxed. He didn't have any headaches or highs; he was just in a sleepy relaxed state.

I was being overly protective, and friends were dividing into the ones who supported me 100 per cent and the ones who told us to stop the treatment with this oil.

Chemo and radiation would have made him sickly, ill, and weak, his hair and teeth falling out. He would have felt dreadful, I wonder if they would have considered this normal My friends reactions showed me how ingrained these "norms" were in everyone's mind—they simply believed that cancer was to be treated with chemo and that chemo made people sick and that was the way it was supposed to be.

## Monday, 13 May

It felt amazing to go to the gym today with Perry for a circuit class. He took a half gram last night and decided to try leaving it until afternoon and evening and splitting the dose in two. He managed a full hour of circuit training. His coordination was a little off, and he was very tired, but it felt great to be doing something normal again.

I found that, when I wrote in my journal, I wrote to release some stress. It allowed me to express everything without having to stop and think about what to write.

In addition, I was getting an incredible amount of support from the friends I'd met on the Internet who was going through or had already gone through the process of taking cannabis oil and cured them. I needed them more now than ever, as I was way out of my league and away from my usual surroundings. As I revisited their blogs or web pages and saw posts from them, I felt at home, comfortable, renewed, uplifted, inspired, and transformed again. They had all been my saviours and were always ready with some encouraging words.

I'd felt such depths of despair and sadness, and yet now right at this very moment, I felt such an inner peace. I knew that meant we were on the right track to healing.

Whenever someone suggested that we consider chemo along with this medicine, I felt extremely drained. It meant clearly, the person making this suggestion hadn't looked at the information I had given them. I knew people were vocalizing their suggestions and objections purely out of concern, but I couldn't understand why, if they felt compelled to express concerns about the effects of the medicine, they wouldn't first endeavour to educate themselves about it. After all, the oil was simply making him sleep more.

Didn't an old wives' tale have it that sleep was the best medicine to heal the body?

I'd learned to open my mind, so the many people who were curing their own illnesses naturally could inspire me, and I felt I was on a path of something very big.

All truths are easy to understand once they are discovered; the point is to just discover them.

## Wednesday, May 15

Yesterday, we decided that Perry should try taking all the medicine at night so he could just sleep it off. So today he hadn't had any yet and was back to normal. We went to the gym. He was driving and conversing as normal.

He was still a little tired and took an hour nap at 4.00 p.m. This was much better, as soon he would need to get back to work, while continuing to get his dosage up to a gram a day while functioning as normally as possible.

## Friday, 17 May

Two weeks into taking the medicine, Perry had still only managed to get his dosage to just over half a gram a day. He'd told me he'd lost his confidence. And I was very worried about him, as his personality was really changing. He wasn't his usual lively self and he seemed lost.

I wrote yet again to the supplier, and she told me that Perry sounded like he was really stoned. She suggested that he take a smaller amount of the medicine. Her recommendation was based purely on her perceptions of how people were responding to each batch of oil and her understanding of science, coupled with what I'd shared about Perry and our life.

Her advice was to cut the dosage back and take it for longer. As long as it was in his system, there was a 70 per cent chance it was working. If he were dying, she would say something different. But he wasn't; he was repairing.

## 18 May

I felt as if I was drowning in all this responsibility, and I wanted my husband back! I missed him so much, and yet, he was right here with me. It was as if his very soul had left him.

Yesterday I tried the oil myself to see what he was dealing with! By now, I was putting it into capsules for him at half-gram doses so he could just take it at night and sleep off the effects. It was all over my fingers when I finished, so I thought I would just taste it. I took only the smallest amount.

After about forty minutes, I started feeling quite strange, and by an hour later, I felt very strange—sort of like my brain was expanding in my head. It wasn't a bad headache; I had just been made aware that it was there. Then I felt a little drunk.

I didn't tell Perry I'd taken it. We were going out to an art exhibition, and while I was drying my hair, it was as if I was watching myself from a distance, sort of an out-of-body experience.

When we were at the exhibition, a friend came over to talk. She must have thought both Perry and I were drunks who had nothing to say! I couldn't think of anything to say except, "I need a drink."

I was utterly embarrassed, and I felt claustrophobic with so many people there, all of whom seemed to be talking very rapidly, especially the friend who'd come over. She kept talking to me, and I couldn't take anything in or think of what to say back to her. I really was on a bad trip (not that I knew what a good trip was). I just wanted to get away. I was experiencing paranoia—sure that everyone was looking at me.

I screamed internally and thanked God I didn't have to take the oil I felt so bad for Perry.

I was very glad I'd been documenting everything so that I could share this with others who decided to take this route. No one had documented the effect the oil had on him or her. In all of the testimonials I'd found the writer said only that he or she'd taken it and it had cured them.

I wrote to my friend again and told her I'd tried the oil. I explained what had happened. She got back to me with this message:

> You got high, sister!!! That's the DMT releasing in your brain. It actually is quite magnificent if you can ride the wave, but you two are super sober, and I am sure it is not a good match for either of you. I can't take it. I never take it. I'm not ill. We don't need it. Not really laughing; more admiring that you were willing to try it!! You are one super cool woman! So happy you are in my life!!!

## 22 May

It was my fifty-fourth birthday today, and I knew instinctively that designer handbags, a flashy car, and the ability to look good first thing in the morning wasn't going to cut the mustard anymore. I had learned so much over this last year, especially, as the old saying goes, that "everything happens for a reason". I wanted to share what I'd learned.

The journey we'd been on had taught me to have faith, not to be afraid to try something new, not to let life just happen to me, to take scary risks, to get real (not just transactional) friends, to laugh till it hurts, to exercise till it hurts, to love, to give, to help others and campaign for what I believe in. Some of the best lessons we learn are learned at the worst times of our lives. But the biggest lesson I'd learned had to do with what really mattered and what didn't! So all in all, this past year had been an amazing year. Happy birthday to me!

## 27 May

Perry was tolerating two-thirds of a gram each night now and waking up alert. But he was still a little slow in his thinking later in the day. He no longer needed to sleep in the day and had been working from home for a week now.

## 29 May

Well, it had almost been four weeks now. I wasn't too homesick. As the old saying goes, "Home is where the heart is." The only thing that was worrying me was that Perry's entire personality had changed. He was no longer bubbly and lively. He got by and could function normally. He wasn't high in the day, but he was a little numbed. He didn't joke like he always did, and he was quite happy doing nothing.

I was worried he couldn't do his job properly while he was under this influence of the oil. But he said the workload wasn't so bad at the moment.

I had to wake him in the mornings now and keep waking him until he finally got up. This was so unlike him. He usually only needed six hour sleeps and was very alert and happy in the mornings. I missed him so much.

## 6 June

Last night, Perry took a full dose of medicine for the first time—one gram in a large capsule all at the same time around 8.00 p.m., so that by the time the effects took place, he could go to bed and sleep it off. I had to wake him at 8.00 this morning and again at 8.30 to get him up. We went to an exercise class, but his coordination was not good. We left after forty-five minutes, as I could see he was struggling.

He was more confused today than normal and completely got things mixed up. It was all beginning to get to me now. I would rather not talk to him, as he seemed like he wasn't listening. I knew it was the medicine, but I was getting really stressed.

## 10 June

I had a very stressful few days. A member of Perry's family had been trying to get him to stop taking this medicine. She'd gone to see another member of the family to ask for backup to come to us both and plead with us to stop this medicine. Instead he had told us what had been requested of him.

The negativity got to me for a while, but we were back on track now. It had been dealt with, and ultimately, I understood where this family member was coming from. But she quite clearly hadn't researched the information I'd sent her, or she would know that nothing would change our minds now. Perry and I told her that, if she didn't support our decision, she needed to stay away ultimately it was our decision and ours alone.

Would anyone be so quick to ask us to stop chemo or radiation if this were the route we were on?.

He would be much worse off if we'd taken that route. It was very hard to have to deal with all of this on top of everything else I was dealing with, and this negativity knocked me back for a few days. But I was glad to say that I was okay and back to my old self again.

Perry was doing so much better now and had been on a full dose of one gram for almost a week now. He was less confused and more awake. He came with me to an hour of circuit training. He struggled a bit, and his fitness had declined since he started taking this medicine. He was slower to react to what the instructor was telling him to do, but he did what he could and left after fifty minutes.

## 14 June

Perry had been on a full dose for eight days now and was tolerating it much better. He'd been waking up earlier and sleeping soundly. He was less groggy in the morning and certainly looked less lethargic. He didn't need to sleep in the day, and he seemed more alert in conversation. He had less memory loss, and his concentration was much higher.

It seemed like he'd managed to get to where he could take the oil without it affecting his daily routine too much. He was driving the car well and worked all day from home. He held conference calls and managed his time much better now. He did seem to have less of an appetite now and said things didn't taste right. His senses of smell and hearing were also heightened.

## 15 June

He managed to wake up alone today, without me having to wake him. He seemed more alert and even asked me if I wanted breakfast for the first time in a very long while.

Witnessing the stark changes in my husband's personality had been very hard. He'd always put me first, but this medicine seemed to have changed his personality for a while. He seemed numb to every emotion, completely indifferent neither happy nor sad and not caring much about anything. But slowly, he was becoming who he'd always been—caring and considerate.

The Journey we'd undergone ever since Perry's diagnosis hadn't been easy on either of us. But now more than ever, I wanted to inspire people. I wanted them to say, "because of you, we didn't give up." Being able to look up to others who inspired me to carry on and showed me the light within myself that enabled me to do so was fantastic.

I believed enlightenment to be the complete uncovering of the truth and the eradication of what we thought to be the truth. I just wanted to pay this back and encourage people to know that, if they found themselves in a situation like ours, then they were the only ones who had the power to change things for themselves. It had slowly but surely occurred to me that people who accomplished the most in this life rarely sat back and just let things happen to them.

## 17 June

Things definitely seemed better during the days, and Perry was able to work well from home. But his personality was still different; he wasn't as fun loving as he used to be. He told me often that he felt like he had no confidence, and he'd lost desire to go out to visit friends to chat, as he couldn't think of anything to talk about. He would answer them, but he wouldn't get involved in a proper conversation with anyone other than for his work.

At least we were more than halfway through the treatment now, and it hadn't caused any pain or suffering at all. I was still missing the old Perry, but I was glad that, at the moment, my family and friends who cared surrounded us. Perry's family were being a little less vocal about what we were doing and I owe that to his Brother's wife who was 100% behind what we were doing.

## 20 June

Perry had been getting more tolerant to the medicine every day. He'd been working each day and seemed to be making idle chatter more often.

His appetite had really slowed down though, and he would need to eat a little more to keep up his weight, as he was still avoiding all sugar, white flour, rice, pasta, and red meats. He'd done very well, sticking to this diet for over a year. It was a complete lifestyle change, not a diet.

I was helping so many others with my journaling of this oil. The oil makers themselves had asked me to share this information, as there was nothing else similar out there. I'd also been in touch with a few people who were making documentaries and were interested in our story. Our journey certainly would help others, and I was very proud to be able to give a little back.

## 27 June

We had just over two more weeks of full dose left, and the end couldn't come quick enough. I wanted my lovely man back beside me in more ways than one. He wasn't the same person he'd been before the medicine. He looked very well, and he wasn't in pain, but the effect it had on him was so great. He was just so quiet and calm, and it was as if all the essence that made him that special person I loved had left him.

## 8 July

We had five more days left of the medicine now, and nothing had changed, other than Perry seemed to be getting quieter. He was also losing a great deal of weight. He had lost four kilograms while taking this medicine, so a total of thirteen kilograms for the year.

But I had to say that he looked remarkably well and so much younger. His skin looked fresh, he looked like the clock had turned back fifteen years.

Still he wasn't his normal bubbly self, and I couldn't wait now for all of this to be over. He was getting paranoid about his job and was eager to get back to normality. He was also talking a lot more about the future and making plans for if anything were to happen to him. He was very worried and eager to find out if the oil had worked.

We booked our tickets home for 23 July, two weeks and a day away—it wouldn't be long now.

## 10 July

Today I received an amazing email from our doctor in the Middle East. It was great that my intuition had led me to him and we'd changed doctors when we had. He was obviously happy to co-doctor Perry so we could find out what we needed to know without causing him any harm.

## 13 July

The day before yesterday, Perry took his last dose of the medicine. It was the largest dose he'd taken since he'd started this treatment. The capsules had leaked, so just over half a gram was in each capsule. He'd taken two. He wasn't making sense all day yesterday. He looked in control, but he was a conversation behind everyone else, so what he was saying didn't make sense to anyone.

Getting through the sixty grams in a ten-week period had been really hard. But at last it was over now, and hopefully we could get back to normal.

Last night, Perry said he had difficulty sleeping, as he didn't have any oil to take. I supposed it would take time before the oil was out of his system. He was really worried his full brain capacity wouldn't be restored; he felt very subdued and lacked confidence.

I wanted my husband back so very much. I was feeling really lonely.

Maybe Perry had taken the medicine too quickly, but we'd had no choice but to do it all in a short time; we'd simply had only twelve weeks to come to England, rent a house, and spend time with family. And I was very grateful that we'd managed to do all of this.

We would leave for the Middle East again in just over a week. Hopefully, this would be enough time to get all the oil out of his system. He'd get back onto his strict diet, and then we'd go to the doctor for a cystoscopy so we could see if the treatment has worked.

## 15 July

Perry today told me he didn't feel well. He was quite agitated and anxious. He felt he needed to get back to his work. Thoughts were flooding his brain as if he were on speed. I thought this must be a withdrawal symptom, so I wrote once again to our supplier in California to ask for advice. I was really worried. He never told me he felt unwell, but he was running around and looked very nervous.

## 18 July

Things were really hard even though Perry had finished the medicine. I realized he probably wouldn't be okay until he'd had the test to check, to see if the medicine had killed the cancer. He was so full of stress now. He hadn't been this way the whole duration of the year that we'd been doing alternative treatments.

It seemed the medicine was very strong and stopping it completely had taken its toll. Everything came flooding back too quickly. He was overthinking things now and full of anxiety. He had never been a worrier. I decided it was withdrawal symptoms, and I didn't think the fact that this medicine had rendered him completely impotent the entire time he was taking it had helped.

He started worrying the impotency and all the changes might be permanent, but I was sure he would be okay as the medicine slowly left his system.

While his appetite had increased at first, once he'd gotten on the full dose, it had declined so drastically that he'd lost an additional four kilograms. He had begun to look drawn now, and the skin on his face had begun to look a little saggy. I was worried myself now. I hoped to God that we would get the all clear on the third of August so I could document the great news to encourage others to finish the treatment. But it wasn't easy at all.

I was glad that I could warn others what to expect though. When I researched withdrawal from marijuana, I learned that it would take up to three weeks to get out of his system and those three weeks were very uncomfortable. He would have anxiety, panic attacks, and mood swings.

He wasn't nice to be around; seeing him panicky and unsure of himself was scary. It didn't help that the Company he worked for had just handed him Tunisia and France to look after, along with Egypt, the Middle East, and India.

I told him he had to take the rest of the week off as sick days. He couldn't work with his brain so overloaded. I was beginning to worry that he'd have a total breakdown if he didn't unwind and relax. I booked him in for a massage and a sauna this afternoon, to help him relax and detox this strong medicine from his body.

## 24 July

We arrived safely back home today. Perry had really suffered since coming off the oil. Thanks to a radio station dedicate to cannabis medicine, I'd been in touch with a few people who'd helped me. I spoke with a cannabis scientist, as well as with moviemaker, Christian Laurette, who'd made *Run from the Cure: The Rick Simpson Story* and was in the process of making *Run from the Cure 2*.

Because I felt so strongly about getting the word out that people who are diagnosed with cancer have options, I had already donated to the movie's production cost. This was a message people needed to hear.

I shared all my concerns about withdrawal and enumerated the effects the medicine had had on my husband's personality, explaining that I couldn't find any documentation or help with these concerns. The panel listened and helped by suggesting other medicine my husband could take in place of the oil, explaining that, as with every medicine, cannabis oil should be come off slowly. I supposed that was common sense. But when you are trying to heal from cancer with a natural cure, you are just so focused on getting the medicine in and taking the full dose.

Christian wrote to me after the show and said this:

> I can't thank you enough.
>
> I am so happy your husband is doing better.
>
> Thanks for your contribution to the movie and for the info! I will mention withdrawal because of your story.

I had sent my journal to Christian and hoped that he read it. If he did mention withdrawal because of our story, at least I would have done some small part to bring this to others' attention. I also gave him the painting, "Taking Control", for my book cover. I offered it to him so he could auction it and use the proceeds to help get the film out to the public.

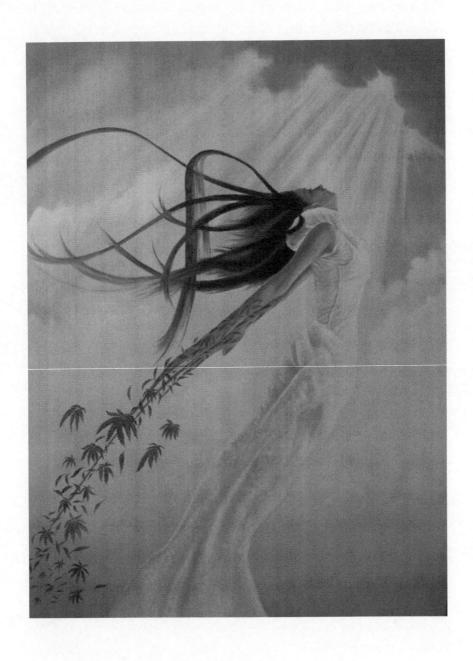

# CHAPTER 9

## DISSAPOINTMENT

### 3 August

Sitting down, I knew this was going to be hard to write. We'd just returned from the cystoscopy, and I had been so sure the cannabis oil would have cured him completely. Perry and I had put all of our hopes on it, and we'd both endured so much trying to get this medicine and finding a way for him to take it.

It had been a long wait to find out the oil hadn't worked the way we had hoped. I was trying to figure out what to write while my world once again fell apart. I didn't want anyone upset or for anyone to think the oil wouldn't work for him or her. I'd done too much research not to believe it worked. It was just that, at this time, it hadn't worked for us the way we'd hoped.

The doctor told us that Perry now had a tumour that had spread to the prostate and many more in the out-pouching of his bladder. Before he'd taken the oil, he'd had only three small tumours in the out-pouching. The doctor couldn't say whether any of them were muscle invasive or if it had spread elsewhere. He needed an MRI to do this.

He told us he could remove all the tumours with another laser surgery, possibly followed by a round of BCG. He stressed to us both that, if he were in our position, he would go for laser time and time again sooner than having the bladder and prostate removed. He congratulated us on keeping away from such radical surgery, as it surely offered no quality of life. He said we were doing the right thing and that the oil could have kept the tumour from being deeply rooted. He added that the tumours could be superficial, reminding us that he couldn't know with the camera.

It was all just sinking in now. I just wanted to vomit. I hadn't been prepared for this outcome. Now we would have to wait for an MRI to be Okayed by the insurance company before we could even find out whether the tumour was superficial or whether it had spread to other organs. If it had, then there would be nothing we could do. If it hadn't, we could continue to have laser treatments each time the tumours showed up.

The doctor was clearly upset for us, but he continued to tell us not to have the bladder and prostate removed if Perry wanted any quality of life. He said that people could keep doing the laser procedure, even for years, every three months and just live with doing that. It would prevent the tumour from spreading. He said again that what we were doing had helped Perry so far and that we should continue.

I knew I couldn't take much more. I was beside myself with fear. Perry was numb.

# CHAPTER 10
## RENEWED HOPE

### 5 August

First, I needed to write about our great news. We just got back from the surgery, and the MRI had shown that the tumours were all confined to the bladder after all. The muscle wall was still clear of tumours, and the tumour that the doctor had thought was in the prostate wasn't. It was a bladder tumour hanging down towards the prostate. The doctor was sure he could remove them all by laser.

The laser procedure would be early next week, and then we'd go back for follow-ups every three months, and if the tumours grew back, we'd keep repeating the treatment.

The doctor thought that he oil had perhaps kept the cancer from metastasis . . . we had good news once again, and once again I was elated!

### What happened after!

I had been visibly upset before the doctor had even looked at the DVD of the MRI. I'd had to wipe my eyes. I'd been so optimistic this entire time, but I felt defeated and responsible. The doctor had kept reminding me of my previous undying optimism and encouraging me not to stop now. It had made me worse; I'd been inconsolable.

So he'd carried on looking at the CD and explaining everything. Immediately, my mood had changed, and I was happy.

Perry had remained his calm self the entire way through the appointment. But when we got outside and got into the car, he just sat there. He told me his legs were shaking. I changed seats, and we set off. He grabbed an envelope and started blowing into it, as if he was hyperventilating. I couldn't pull over, as I was on a busy road.

Then he started crying and threw up all over the car and me. It was the release of all the worry. I felt so helpless here on our own. I had to ring his boss and tell him the good news and that Perry couldn't come into work today.

Perry's boss understood and congratulated me. He told me to tell Perry to take the week off, saying he realized what a huge burden a man carried when he had something like this hanging over him, all the while holding down a job and worrying about his family. He had been great.

Perry was now sleeping, and all was good once again.

Now that I'd had time to reflect, it seemed like the oil had done a good job of stopping the metastasis. I'd spoken with Jack Kungel (a great guy), who'd cured his own bladder and prostate cancer with diet, alkalizing his body, and using the oil. He advised me about a smoothie I could make for Perry. I would get on that straight away.

I was back to fighting this beast head on again, but boy, I had taken a beating. And so had my beautiful man.

### Wednesday, 14 August

Perry had the laser surgery two days earlier. He stayed in overnight, and came out yesterday. He hadn't experienced any pain and still didn't. He got right back to work. He was lucky to have an amazing surgeon and an office-based job that required no heavy lifting.

Perry seemed very well considering the doctor said he'd removed many tumours. He still believed they were superficial, but we couldn't be sure, as no biopsies had been done.

Our plan now was to speak to the doctor in a week's time about what we were going to do next. We needed to decide whether we were just going to stick with cystoscopies to check inside the bladder every three monthly or whether we were going to do BCG. We needed to look into this further! My feelings now were that we should stick to the alkaline diet he had been on and just go by how he felt. We were still considering him taking the oil as a maintenance dose.

I had so many new friends now who were on this journey with me and offering me so much support. It felt like I always had somebody who was ready to give a little advice, and I no longer felt alone on this journey of healing for my husband.

Perry was also much more involved in all the research now and was actively helping me juice and make his smoothies, which took a long time to prepare. It had taken a lot of worry and work off my shoulders, and I knew now that he was capable of eating and choosing all the foods that would build his immune system for himself without my having to prompt him.

He kept telling me he felt like his body was loaded with oxygen, no doubt a result of all the green juices. They had this effect on his body and made him feel like he did as a young man.

I was so impressed with the way he felt and also with how he kept telling me how well he was and that he wanted to get back to the gym. He told me he would never go back to his old ways of not taking care of himself or eating the way he did. I was full of hope and inspiration once again!

## 20 August

Our visit to the doctor this morning was promising. Perry had an ultrasound scan to check his liver, and all was good—the scan found no inflammation and no obstruction in the bladder either.

The doctor had a DVD of the operation, and we watched about fifteen minutes of his laser surgery. It was amazing! Technology allowed me to see inside my husband's bladder for myself. We didn't have to trust anyone but could see with our own eyes. We discussed our next plans, which were to have another cystoscopy in five weeks' time. If no tumours were emerging, the doctor would then implant the BCG cocktail directly to the bladder and continue to do this once weekly for six weeks and, thereafter, once monthly for six months. This would work to kill any rogue cells, leaving his healthy ones to thrive.

The doctor did say, however, that the cancer had not spread outside the bladder or gone into any lymph nodes. It was all still contained, and his blood tests were all normal. He told us again that what we were doing had almost certainly kept the cancer from spreading and added that Perry looked fresh, happy, and healthy. He did indeed.

## 28 August

Perry played a game of squash for the first time in about ten years last week, but he paid for it with a lot of aches and pains afterwards. He was okay, though, and looking forward to taking this sport up on a regular basis. He seemed to have more energy than he had in such a long while. Maybe I could even take my mind off the fact that he was supposed to be sick.

Still, he had some blood in his urine according to his most recent blood work, but that had only been around ten days after surgery. The doctor had said it was only scar tissue getting released; he told us not to worry about it and to enjoy Perry's newfound energy and zest for life.

## 30 August

We just had some young people (the son and daughter-in-law of one of our friends) round to buy a painting. How amazed they were to see how well Perry looks. When they asked what he'd done to achieve this, we both began to tell our story of refusing chemo, radiation, and surgery.

They wanted to read my journal and were going to begin to change the way they ate and drank and to stop being scared of the word *cancer*. They were on their way to their friends full of our story and a great new topic of conversation. One at a time, the word was getting out!

## 3 Sept

Something wasn't right with Perry. He'd become stressed and snappy all the time lately. He kept telling me that my oil hadn't worked and I was acting like he was already cured. Well, I had to act like he was cured because I had to be positive.

Looking at the positive told me the cancer hadn't spread and Perry looked and felt well; looking at the negative told me the cure on which we'd mistakenly pinned all our hopes had not completely cured him. We'd somehow expected it to be a quick fix, and now I believed that Perry was scared but wouldn't admit it.

I'd spoken to many people who'd used our methods of treatment and they all said they were scared to death. But most of them had had to do their own research, whereas I was the one to do all this research. Perry trusted me to inform him. I was the one who had educated him and myself.

I tried talking to my sister, but she just told me, "He thinks the oil didn't work because it didn't."

I realized I could now only talk to people who had gone through the situation we were facing themselves. And I was so grateful I had that lifeline. I had people who inspired me and made me see that I wasn't the one to blame here. We still had a plan, and as far as I could see, everything was working. Perry was just feeling a little negative right now for some reason.

I spoke at great length with my friend, Jack, who'd cured his own prostate and bladder cancer. He told me he'd had to do the oil treatment seven times before he'd been cured and added that a maintenance dose should be taken for life. Jack had given me the recipe for the pH smoothie that Perry now drank daily.

I believed that it had all has just gotten to be too much for Perry. He threw all his vitamins in the trash this morning and made bacon for the first time in thirteen months. He was rebelling. I didn't nag. I just left the house to figure out what to do.

I spoke to my lifeline, Jack, who was my saviour when I lost the ability to carry on. Jack told me I just had to wait for Perry to see that I wasn't the enemy. He asked me how many wives could do what I had done for their men. Jack told me Perry was the one who needed an attitude adjustment, and I needed a break from looking after him. I had been by his side since July of last year when he'd first been diagnosed—at every hospital trip, every doctor's visit, and every scan and examination.

I did need a break. Jack was right. I decided to go see my beautiful granddaughters in England, and hopefully, I'd be missed.

## 5 Sept

All was calm in the house again. Perry Skyped with Jack as he'd suggested, and they'd chatted alone about everything they both were feeling. Jack was amazing and helped Perry so much. Perry told him he'd never even eaten the bacon; he'd thrown it in the trash when he'd retrieved his vitamins. He was just feeling despondent that he couldn't raise his pH level. He was also worried about the oncoming BCG treatment, but Jack talked him through it all step by step and explained that it was a good thing to do. He also told him that his own wife wouldn't even listen to him about taking this alternative route and that he had an amazing ally in me.

Perry was sorry that he'd been negative for a few days, but he was back on track now and looking at his diet again to raise his pH levels. We added a few more things to his smoothie and took a bit of the fruit out to see if that would work. He also added a half teaspoon of bicarbonate of soda to the drink, and he would need to take potassium while taking this.

## 7 August

Jack had been such a godsend to both Perry and me over the past month. He gave his time so freely to help people like myself understand what needed to be done. Although I'd researched for many months now, it is always nice to have a mentor to turn to when things get tough. And Jack had helped Perry so much.

What follows is Jack Kungel's amazing story of his healing in his own words:

I had eight surgeries. I have bilateral carpel tunnel, bilateral ulnar nerve entrapment, two torn rotator cuffs, two torn bicep tendons, torn cartilage in the meniscus tendon and the cruciate ligament in my right knee, and a hernia. This happened when some steel was falling and I caught it to keep my feet from being crushed.

For the next twenty years, I threw up two to three times a day from the medication. I lost my teeth because the stomach acid ate them. I have four permanently damaged ribs from puking and permanent nerve damage in my upper girdle and the hernia from puking (it consistently and persistently feels like someone is stabbing me with a knife).

I had 543 visits to therapy and about forty cortisone injections into my shoulders to keep my arms mobile, and they were not successful. I had my right knee scoped sixteen times.

I was at death's door due to pharmaceutical toxicity from the drugs my doctors had me on. My body was in convulsions from reactions to everything.

I did some research and found cannabis. I stopped every single medication I was on and just *ingested cannabis*—three grams daily ground up in capsules and three cookies. My life has made a complete turnaround as I result of ingesting cannabis

Since 1991 when I got injured at work, I was on the following medication:

120 mg oxyContin
30 mg morphine
30 mg Toradol
4 Tylenol 4
150 mg Amitriptaline
200 mg Celebrex
2,000 mg metformin
15 mg lipator
15 mg Clonazepam

In addition, I took 20 mg of Zantac for acid reflux from the medication.

Since I began ingesting this plant three years ago just for pain, these were the side effect of cannabis:

1. My pain went from a 9.5 every day to a 3.
2. I stopped throwing up after twenty years (within a day!) and have not gotten sick since.
3. I could sleep for the first time in twenty years, as the feeling that my arms had been ripped off was relieved. (*My god this was unbelievable.*)

4. I could lift my arms over my head. It was uncomfortable, but I could do it

5. I had a gradual weight loss over three years of forty-six pounds.

6. My blood sugar was lowered to normal range.

7. I haven't had a cold or flu in three years (and haven't had a flu shot).

8. The fissure cracks in my feet that would bleed and need medical attention went away. They are soft!

9. The moles and warts and skin tags are falling off my skin

10. The diabetic nerve pain is gone.

★   ★   ★

*Then came bladder cancer!* Specifically, I was diagnosed with adenocarcinoma of the bladder.

Here's the best explanation I could find: "These tumours arise in patients who have a long history of cystitis; glandular cystitis frequently is associated with this lesion. These tumours resemble colonic carcinoma, and most have invaded into muscle at the time of initial diagnosis. These tumours frequently produce mucin, with the signet cell variant being rare and particularly aggressive. Primary adenocarcinoma of the bladder is treatable and potentially curable with radical cystectomy or pelvic exenteration.

This type of cancer travels with the blood. I had my first surgery in February 2011. The surgeons removed a large tumour and these bleeding lesions from the bladder walls. I was told then that the bladder needed to be removed. My prostate was also involved, and I had the TURP ( Transurethral Resection of the prostate procedure. My doctors gave me six BCG Bacillus Calmette-Guérin) treatments. BCG is an injection of the tuberculosis virus to induce an immune system attack on the bladder to fluff all its cells.

I had a reaction to the BCG and got acid burns. My body was acidic, and the reaction was a rash all over my body that I had for over two yrs. I couldn't go out in the sun, and if I sweated, it got worse.

I started on the oil, made butter, ate it, baked with it, and got as much cannabis it into me as I could and then stopped.

But the cancer came back! That's when I learned how *acidic* I was. I checked my pH level, and I was at 3.5—the danger zone and an environment that cancer loves. So I started with the Baking soda and molasses cancer protocol. This helped to raise my pH.

But I needed more to give my body the food it needed to fight this cancer. So I started to make a smoothie in which every ingredient would raise the body's alkalinity. This smoothie has brought my pH levels to 8.5 to 9. And it will do this in just a few days. In addition, I stopped all sugar intake because *cancer feeds on sugar*!

Here's the recipe for the alkaline smoothie:

1 tsp sunflower seeds
1 tsp pumpkin seed
12 almonds
2 Brazil nuts
4 walnut halves
2 tbsp hemp hearts
1 tsp flax seed
> (Grind these first and then add them to mixture. I use the Nutra Bullet and it works awesome!)

Spinach
1 Brussels sprout
3 sprigs asparagus
Kale
2 radishes
Broccoli
parsley

1 slice fresh pineapple

1 1/2 inch slice lemon, peel and all

2 strawberries

4 blackberries

12 blueberries

3 chunks watermelon

4 chunks cantaloupe

1 kiwi

> Then add a cup of juice. I use carrot. You can add whatever liquid you prefer, as long as it's healthy.

## 8 Sept

Today, we booked in to have Perry's cystoscopy and insertion of BCG on Tuesday, 18 September. His visit to the doctor this morning was due to the fact that his pH test strip showed he had too much protein. The doctor said this could indicate his levels were now too alkaline. We had to wait for a culture test, which would take three days.

I felt like we needed to keep him alkaline, and we were doing so well. Now this was showing that, perhaps, we were overdoing it.

As I was adding new paintings to my art site, I realized that, for the last year, all I'd been painting has been related to my feelings and my journey with cancer. My latest was a self-portrait—well a sort of a fantasy style self-portrait of a woman standing on the edge of a cliff and almost falling off. She is smiling, as she has no fear; she has surrendered herself to the will of the universe. This has been how I've felt most of the time. I try not to let negativity in; I am, most of the time, focused and strong. I don't let the noise of others' opinions drown out my own inner voice. And most importantly, I have the courage to follow my own heart and intuition. They somehow already know what I truly need. Everything else is secondary.

I looked through my art page over the last year and saw comments I'd written and couldn't even remember doing so. This journey had consumed me, and yet, it had awakened such an inner strength.

Inspiration is a message in a bottle from me, a window into my other world; it comes when I least expect it. When it gets too much for me, I paint.

## 12 September

Today, Perry flew to England to visit our sons. It would just be a four-day visit. The last time they'd seen him, he hadn't been himself; he'd been under the influence of a very strong medicine called cannabis oil. They were both worried; he hadn't been very communicative and he'd looked like he had lost too much weight.

This visit would be nice, allowing them both to see their father and feel reassured that he was better. Not being able to see him regain his weight and his mental awareness must have been very worrying for them.

Perry's main goal at the time had been to get back to his job in the place we called home. We had both been through so much as we'd tried to get the ninety—day treatment out of the way, and we had pinned so much hope on it being a silver bullet cure.

It hadn't worked out that way, and now we realized that Perry would need to take the oil for the rest of his life. We had both done a lot of soul searching to come to the conclusion that we needed to get this medicine and bring it here so he could take the maintenance dose.

I'd stayed behind, and I was so nervous waiting for his safe and speedy return.

A friend told me today that she could see that I was drained. I was—by this thing called cancer and the risks we'd had to undertake just to get a plant-based medicine. This journey had changed our lives. I realized and confessed to her that I had forgotten how to smile for the sake of just smiling.

Perry's diagnosis and everything that followed had changed me. I didn't even remember who I was anymore—what I liked to read or what music I liked to listen to. My reading material changed at once from *Fifty Shades of Grey* to *World without Cancer*. I had forgotten what brought me joy. I spent my spare time looking at videos of people who had cured their own Cancers or speaking with people on Facebook about this subject. I helped people looking for answers.

I didn't know how to get back to just being me. How could I, when I had learned so much that could change the way we as a society look at cancer. And even if Perry were to get the all clear, I would be watching for its return every three months.

I missed the easiness we'd once had together. I missed our playfulness, and I missed myself. I missed simply feeling no worries, just wrapped in the pleasant and blissful companionship that had become our marriage. I'd forgotten my old dreams. They were no longer of importance, and nothing else seemed to matter.

I now had new dreams, new goals. I had to learn more about this new me and what she felt for others who'd been diagnosed with cancer. I now had this mission in life—to find out whether cancer could be cured with a plant-based medicine and the proper nutrition, without the standard protocol of chemo, radiation, and surgery. I also had a mission to help others see their way through all the heartache of first finding out they had cancer and then feeling they had no hope to finding someone to understand and guide them to look at their options. I wanted to help them see they could investigate their options, that an endless amount of research was available to them, and that they could and should listen to their own intuition when it came to the treatments that are on offer

## 15 September

"Courage is contagious. When someone brave takes a stand, the spines of others are often stiffened." Billy Grahem

I'd learned so much in the past fourteen months; I'd learned that courage is not without fear but the triumph over it; that bravery is to be able to conquer that fear; and that the hardest choices in life sometimes aren't between what's right and wrong but between what's right and what needs to be done. In any moment after diagnosis, the worst thing you can do is nothing.

## 16 Sept

Yesterday was the longest day of my life. I was pacing the floor at the airport waiting for the time to pass and I nervously awaited my husbands' return. I was sweating and almost throwing up in the waiting area. The plane was delayed, adding to my anxiety, which was building by the minute. I had felt sick to my stomach all day.

Perry arrived safe and sound, and I was so proud of him and of the fact that we were both brave enough to do what needed to be done.

## 17 Sept

Today's doctor visit showed no return of any tumours in the bladder, so we decided to go ahead with a treatment the doctor had offered that would complement our alternative approach to healing with nutrition and alternative medicines.

Perry had his first of six weekly BCG treatments. Hopefully, help prevent the cancer from coming back in the bladder lining, and it would also reduce the risk of it becoming invasive. It's usually given when there is a high risk that the cancer will come back and grow into the bladder muscle (become invasive).

Perry was home and resting. The procedure had been uncomfortable, but he was happy to know that something we were doing was definitely working.

He had to lie down for two hours, turning every ten minutes to coat the bladder on all sides with the medicine.

He was back to work now, so we knew this treatment wouldn't disrupt him too much for the next six weeks.

## 19 September

I was smiled out, talked out, quipped out, and socialized out. I needed the weight of mortal silences or maybe just the lonely beach in the morning to get back into myself. I needed a holiday!

## 24 September

The second BCG went well today. Perry wasn't experiencing any side effects from the treatment, and he back to work within two hours. We were beginning to settle down now, in the knowledge that at least the cancer was under control and he wasn't getting sick or feeling ill in any way.

We were beginning to see that we could live with this invisible thing called cancer. The doctors had told us it was terminal, but we were seeing no signs of this whatsoever. We just knew he had it and that he had to carry on with all the alternative treatments we'd chosen. This was what was keeping him well.

## 28 September

We were starting to go out a lot more lately. It had been a full year of research and not much time for anything else. We were forgetting to live our lives, and now that we'd managed to get through this year with flying colours, we were back in the world we loved and knew. We were meeting new friends and having fun at last.

## 2 October

It was now fourteen months since diagnosis. We were both still quite fragile, but I wanted to write my thoughts on how proud I was of the way my husband was handling everything. He was a truly amazing man. He carried on like he didn't have a care in the world. He'd been sailing through his recent BCG treatments, which he took weekly on the same day he saw a personal trainer to help him get his new body back into building muscle mass. He was just as considerate as he'd always been, and he still remembered to buy me flowers and say, "Good morning, beautiful," to me every single day. I saw him watching me a lot.

He didn't ever talk to me of his fears. Neither of us ever talked about what if. We were both too tuned into the fact that he was healing and that he hadn't had one day in pain or sickness in the entire fourteen months since diagnosis.

We may have had a few disagreements, but love had not failed us. We'd made it through all of the other difficult times, and we would make it through this one too. I loved him so much, and I knew we were so much stronger today than we had been a year ago.

I couldn't express how grateful I was for the way he was handling everything. I knew it wasn't easy for him, and I needed to tell him more how proud I was of him for sticking to this lifestyle change, which was so hard to do. I could never imagine my life without him in it. He was so strong, loving, and successful in everything he did. I prayed that God would keep him safe and keep giving him the strength, wisdom, and patience to carry on, seeing this process of healing through to the end.

It would be our thirty-fourth wedding anniversary in December, and I looked forward to all the years we still had in our future.

# 4 November

Perry had completed his six treatments now and he was tolerating the BCG really well, with only a couple of days of being uncomfortable after each treatment. He'd now had a break of two weeks from the treatments, and tomorrow he had to go for a cystoscopy to check to see whether any new tumours had formed or whether we had kept them at bay.

In addition, we had a very interesting conversation with the anaesthetist who would look after Perry tomorrow during his cystoscopy. She told him he looked amazing and that all his vital signs were in peak condition, including his blood pressure and oxygen levels. She asked about his history and sat and listened to me telling her all we'd done to save his bladder. I told her all about the digestive enzymes having to work so hard to digest processed food that they were no longer able to do the job of healing the body, which led to the immune system being compromised. It was such a miracle of nature that, given the right nutrition, our bodies could heal themselves of most diseases, including cancer.

All modern medicine ever attempts to do is mask the experiential symptoms of a disease without ever holistically healing the origin of the condition itself and, thereby, without healing the disease, often causing even more harm to the patient through chemical medicines and invasive surgical procedures.

In most people today, the immune system is often already highly compromised through a poor diet and lifestyle, environmental toxins, and other factors.

Natural is always best, and in the context of the immune system, this means a natural, healthy, and effective diet.

By far, the best foods and drinks to maintain a balance and, therefore the immune system are foods containing no added chemicals.

The anaesthetist told us she's met one particular doctor who said to her many months ago that all degenerative illnesses could be cured with the right kinds of food, especially plant-based foods. We were there for a ten-minute appointment, and we came out two hours later. She was amazed at how well and how young Perry looked. She also told me that I was an inspiration and that he was a very lucky man to have such a dedicated wife.

I had to stop short of telling her about the cannabis oil. Hopefully one day I will openly tell people about it.

## 5 November

Today, Perry had the cystoscopy to check for any new tumours growing. The doctor promised to send someone out to me to let me know before they started using the laser if new tumours had been found.

I waited fifteen minutes before a nurse I now knew very well came out with a big smile on her face to let me know that there were no new tumours and everything looked nice and clear. I hugged her tightly. I was elated. All our hard work was at last paying off.

My husband was still sleeping and didn't know the good news yet.

When he came back to the hospital room, I told him he had no catheter and his doctor had found no trace of new tumours. We were both delighted. Something was working!

The doctor came in and let us know that he had seen a little swelling in two areas but nothing like before, and that could simply be irritation from the BCG. He said he'd decided to laser that area just to be safe and that he suggested Perry now have six weekly intervals of BCG, as it has worked well for him with no side effects.

I let everyone know, and I was exquisitely happy for the first time in such a long while. I felt at ease and very tired all of a sudden. Perhaps it was a body reaction telling me I could relax a little now.

I needed to let everyone know that all this hard work was worth it in the end. My husband still had his bladder and his life. He was healthier than he had been ten years ago, and we would continue on this journey and get back to them soon. What I most wanted to convey to people was this: Please, if you take anything from our story, know that there is another way; you do have a choice when you are faced with a dreadful diagnosis. Research and give 100 per cent to finding a natural cure and you will see the change that you can achieve as your body does what it is designed for—healing itself

# CHAPTER 11

## LOOKING BACK

What a year 2013 had been for us as a family. We'd learned so much, such as how to be happy, or travel, or going forward—even though all our plans seemed to be fading away in the face of other problems— even though suddenly we had to focus on just trying to survive. We now were faced with tasks wed never imagined—obtaining an illegal substance to take as a medicine, cooking and eating a completely new diet of only healthy foods, and using most of our savings in the process. During this year, I'd been shown what truly rich rewards could be reaped from love and determination and that, in every cloud, there is a silver lining and out of every crisis comes an opportunity. It was a year chalk full of dysfunction; heartache; bewilderment; and, at times, fear and anguish. Yet it had also been filled with so much love from family and special friends. We had seen a great deal of love, tenderness, compassion, and some hilarious moments that would go down in history through the writing of *Taking Control* and journaling our progress with using alternative medicine. I hoped to carry on writing, as I'd found it so cathartic.

It had been a year in which I believed I'd grown so much spiritually and learned to trust my instincts above all else. I had become at peace now with the word *cancer* and what it truly meant, and I considered that peace a blessing that I could now pass on to others.

This past year, I'd reached out to so many others for help myself, and I'd felt overwhelming gratitude for the people who'd given of themselves so selflessly once they knew the truth about what alternative medicine could do for the body. I could never find the right words to tell you how much gratitude and love I felt for them.

## 18 January

Tomorrow, Perry would have his next cystoscopy to check to see whether new tumours were developing. We'd had a three-month reprieve.

To date, I'd shared my journal with so many desperate people looking for a gentler way to heal their bodies. I'd joined a website with over 10,000 people looking into cannabis oil as an alternative treatment for many diseases. Many times, I'd shared my thoughts on this page about a total lifestyle change, which includes, first and foremost, nutrition and vitamin therapy and then the oil. Many people were interested in our story, purely because I documented everything and had found out that, not only can you take time to do some research, but you can also turn the clock back ten years at the same time you are healing your own body with this gentle method.

I'd shared my journal many times with desperate people who couldn't wait for me to publish what I'd discovered. And I'd received an outpouring of gratitude for keeping this journal and sharing our story. Each and every person who had read it had sent me an email of thanks, which I proudly kept in a file to look back on and inspire me to carry on trying to do what I could to let people know that there is another way to treat cancer and that the government does know about it and is keeping it from us.

I planned to continue journaling Perry's health for the next forty-two weeks, when I could actually say he was at the five-year survival mark, which by traditional treatment would count as the marker to say he is cured.

★   ★   ★

The last few days hadn't been easy on either of us, as Perry's cystoscopy would let us look inside his bladder. We could find nothing, or we could see signs that, again, the cancer was rearing its ugly head.

But what I did know was that we were already past the mark the doctors had predicted that he would die if he did not remove his bladder and prostate and take six weeks of intensive chemo and radiation. And we had done none of those horrifying treatments.

Needless to say, we were feeling a little more confident that he would survive now. But it didn't stop the apprehensions that inevitably crept into our hearts and minds about a week before each test or MRI.

The Government, Doctors and scientists keep asking for evidence, and evidence is exactly what all these success stories are. I hope to one day be part of such evidence as it's presented to scientists, with all of our documentation and biopsy slides, all the MRIs and doctors' reports. I want to demonstrate how the doctors initially used terms like *severe* and *aggressive* to frighten us into doing what they said.

Gathering success stories is extremely difficult because of one thing—the government's failure to act; and that is a true shame. From 1850 to 1937, cannabis was used as the prime medicine for more than 100 separate illnesses and diseases in the US "pharmacopeia" (though most of this information was destroyed). And still, the government will not conduct the research and patient trials necessary to get the evidence on cannabis's healing properties. In fact, in 1942, marijuana was removed from US pharmacopeia, therefore, losing its remaining mantle of therapeutic legitimacy.

## 19 January

I sat in the waiting area while Perry was under anaesthetic yet again. The doctor had once more promised to send his nurse out to let me know if he'd spotted any tumours through the cystoscope before he started to laser them off.

I sat, and I prayed like I had never prayed before.

Then just twenty minutes later, both the surgeon and his nurse, who knew me quite well by now—both knew all I had done, that I had written about everything, and how much I loved my husband— walked towards me with sad faces.

I stood waiting to hear bad news when they both burst into big smiles and told me his bladder is clean as a whistle.

Oh my god—we had actually done it. The cystoscopy had shown not even the slightest inflammation—no sign Perry had ever had anything wrong with him.

I couldn't find the words for what I felt at that moment. I had been sitting and praying so hard to God to let this news be so good that people would have to listen—that they would have to see that another way to cure cancer did, in fact, exist. I was crying with joy. I had proof now that what I'd known all along was true—we can live our lives safe in the knowledge that our body can heal itself if we treat it right.

## 20 January

At the doctor's office today, Perry's doctor showed us a video of the inside of Perry's bladder from yesterday's cystoscopy. The doctor was so hyped up and amazed. He told Perry that he had never seen such results before. He also told him that, among the three of us, Perry owed this success to one person—the person writing a book about his success.

He actually had printed a copy of my journal (up to the end of the summer and about 100 pages long) and had it on his desk. He told me he wanted a signed copy! I was so incredibly proud and so happy.

The doctor said he'd write a report for me tomorrow, as he knew I wanted it to finish my book. What a perfect end, to my book—for now anyway.

*   *   *

I will keep writing as so much will be happening, and I won't be able to say that Perry is cured until we've reached the five-year mark. Still, he's had no cancer for the past six months, and that's keeping our spirits up. And he's still doing regular checks every three months. Hopefully by the time five years is up and he is still okay, the world will know more about what I have been harping on about and sharing in my own way for the past year!

## 21 January

I just got the report from the doctor's office. It read, "On 19 January, 2014,

Underwent flexible cystoscopy under GA. This showed absolutely no abnormalities, no recurrent bladder mass."

Thank you all for reading about our journey—our success story. I just know you are smiling with me, and I'm sure some of you are reading this with your mouths open in dis belief. But, wow, what a way to end my journal for the time being.